instructor's manual & testbank to accompany

pediatric NURSING
caring for children

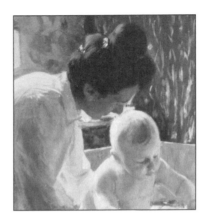

second edition

Instructor's Manual
Mary L. Burke, DNSc, RN
Professor of Nursing
Rhode Island College
Providence, Rhode Island

Testbank
Laurie A. Materna, RN, MSN
Instructor
Milwaukee Area Technical College
Milwaukee, Wisconsin

Appleton & Lange
Stamford, Connecticut

www.appletonlange.com

99 00 01 02 03/ 10 9 8 7 6 5 4 3 2 1

Prentice Hall International (UK) Limited, *London*
Prentice Hall of Australia Pty. Limited, *Sydney*
Prentice Hall Canada, Inc., *Toronto*
Prentice Hall Hispanoamericana, S.A., *Mexico*
Prentice Hall of India Private Limited, *New Delhi*
Prentice Hall of Japan, Inc., *Tokyo*
Simon & Schuster Asia Pte. Ltd., *Singapore*
Editora Prentice Hall do Brasil Ltda., *Rio de Janeiro*
Prentice Hall, *Upper Saddle River, New Jersey*

ISBN 0-8385-8167-6

Acquisitions Editor: David P. Carroll
Designer: Libby Schmitz

PRINTED IN THE UNITED STATES OF AMERICA

CONTENTS

NURSE'S ROLE IN CARE OF THE ILL AND INJURED CHILD: HOSPITAL, COMMUNITY SETTINGS, AND HOME

Chapter Overview

Chapter 1 introduces the numerous roles of the nurse caring for children with health problems and their families in a variety of settings. Using a pediatric perspective, it examines clinical practice roles, the nursing process, care settings, and the contemporary climate for care, including cultural issues, statistics, and health care issues. Legal concepts relating to nursing practice are introduced. The chapter concludes with a discussion of legal and ethical issues encountered in providing health care for children. They include informed consent, conflicting rights of the child and parents, confidentiality, and the Patient Self-Determination Act. Short case studies pose questions for the areas discussed.

Learning Objectives

- Discuss the role of the nurse in pediatric practice.
- List five possible settings for pediatric nursing practice.
- Identify the key elements of family-centered care.
- Describe the impact of a family's culture on the care of a child.
- Interpret the mortality and morbidity statistics for children.
- Discuss how mortality and morbidity statistics can be used in pediatric nursing practice.

- Discuss the impact of research, lifesaving technology, and health care financing on the family and society.
- Outline the benefits of home care for chronically ill children.
- Explain how pediatric nurses assume responsibility and accountability for their practice.
- Summarize the nursing information that must be documented in a patient's record.
- Describe the nurse's role in obtaining informed consent.
- Discuss the ethical decision-making process.

Key Terms

advance directives
assent
continuity of care
continuum of care
critical pathways
emancipated minors
family-centered care
informed consent
mature minors
moral dilemma
morbidity
quality assurance
quality improvement
risk management

Chapter Outline

Role of the Nurse in Pediatrics
  Clinical Practice
    Direct Nursing Care
    Patient Education
    Patient Advocate
    Case Management
  Nursing Process in Pediatric Care
  Settings for Pediatric Nursing Care
Contemporary Climate for Pediatric Nursing Care
  Family-Centered Care
  Culturally Sensitive Care
  Pediatric Health Statistics
  Health Care Issues
    Health Care Technology
    Health Care Financing
Legal Concepts and Responsibilities
  Regulation of Nursing Practice
  Accountability and Risk Management
    Accountability
    Risk Management
Legal and Ethical Issues in Pediatric Care
  Informed Consent
  Child's Rights versus Parents' Rights
  Confidentiality
  Patient Self-Determination Act
  Ethical Issues
    Terminating Life-Sustaining Treatment
    Organ Transplantation Issues

Tables

Overhead Transparencies

Audio-Visual Resources

1. *A Quiet Revolution ... The First Twenty Years*
   Videocassette, 23 minutes
   Source: Association for the Care of Children's Health
2. *The Pediatric Nurse as Teacher*
   Videocassette, 20 minutes
   Source: Medical Electronic Educational Services, Ltd.
3. *Critical Choice*
   Videocassette, 15 minutes
   Source: Pyramid Films
4. *Peace Has Not Been Made: A Case History of a Hmong Family's Encounter with a Hospital*
   Videocassette, 25 minutes
   Source: Rhode Island Office of Refugee Resettlement

Potential Problem Areas for Students

1. Students may have difficulty interpreting mortality and morbidity statistics. Use of an overhead transparancy with graphs of some key statistics could help to focus discussion and identify any problems with comprehension.
2. Students may not recognize the potential conflicts between children's and parents' rights in situations related to informed consent and confidentiality. A handout that lists policies specific to the laws of the state in these situations may be helpful.

Activities to Foster Critical Thinking

A. CLASSROOM ACTIVITIES

1. Show the videotape, "A Quiet Revolution ... The First Twenty Years." Have students identify:
   (a) the major areas of progress in providing psychosocial care for children,

(b) the changing role of the nurse in the field of children's health care,

(c) ways in which nurses could be active in improving health care for children.

2. Present a case study on a child with newly diagnosed diabetes mellitus. Ask students to identify areas of intervention and patient teaching that may be impacted by cultural beliefs and practices.

3. Present statistics on morbidity or mortality for children under the age of 18 years in the state for the last five years. Ask students to:

(a) examine the statistics for trends,

(b) suggest factors that may have caused the morbidity or mortality rates to change, and

(c) suggest policies or specific actions that might reduce these rates.

4. Present a situation of a 16-year-old pregnant girl who comes to the Emergency Room with vaginal bleeding. Ask students to discuss potential issues of confidentiality and conflict between the patient's rights and her parents' rights.

5. Present a case study of a preschool child with a severe abdominal injury and internal bleeding whose parents are Jehovah's Witnesses. Have one group of students argue the legal and ethical issues involved from the viewpoint of the parents and another group argue the perspective of the health care team.

B. CLINICAL ACTIVITIES

1. Have each member of the student group observe or interview a nurse in a different role during the clinical rotation. At a clinical conference, have the students present the key elements of the role they observed, critique its effectiveness, identify barriers to its effectiveness, and suggest ways in which it might be implemented differently.

2. Have students identify the various cultural backgrounds of the children seen that day in the clinical setting. For each culture, have students identify one potential barrier to effective care and suggest an intervention for avoiding or overcoming this obstacle.

3. Have students accompany a staff nurse during the admission of a child to an acute care unit to observe informed consent protocols; have students review the records of their patients to evaluate informed consent procedures that have been implemented.

4. Provide copies of agency policies on informed consent and emergency resuscitation. At a clinical conference, ask students to discuss these as they apply to:

(a) the child,

(b) the parents, and

(c) the responsibilities of the pediatric nurse.

2

GROWTH AND DEVELOPMENT

Chapter Overview

Chapter 2 presents an overview of growth and development from birth through adolescence. It begins with descriptions of the developmental purposes of play, principles of growth and development, factors that influence development and the major developmental theories. The nursing application of each theory is described. The chapter then presents in-depth information specific to each developmental stage. Within each stage, this information is organized into the categories of physical growth and development, cognitive development, play or activities, nutrition, injury prevention, personality and temperament, and communication. The adolescent section includes information on sexuality. Throughout the chapter, tables highlight developmental milestones and present important information in a developmental context.

Learning Objectives

- Describe the general principles of growth and development.
- Apply the theories of Piaget, Erikson, and Freud to children ranging in age from birth to adolescence.
- Identify physical and behavioral milestones that are characteristic of children in each age group.
- Recognize coping strategies used by children and adolescents.
- Describe normal patterns of play exhibited by children.

- List toys that are appropriate for young children.
- Discuss normal nutrition for children in each age group.
- Identify various hazards that can cause injuries to children and adolescents.
- Discuss characteristics of children's communication from birth through adolescence.

Key Terms

accommodation
anticipatory guidance
assimilation
associative play
cephalocaudal development
conservation
cooperative play
defense mechanism
development
dramatic play
expressive jargon
growth
nature
nurture
object permanence
parallel play
proximodistal development
puberty
sensitive periods

Chapter Outline

Physical Growth and Development
Cognitive Development
Play
Nutrition
Injury Prevention
Personality and Temperament
Communication
Principles of Growth and Development
Major Theories of Growth and Development
    Freud's Theory of Psychosexual Development
        Theoretical Framework
        Stages
        Nursing Application
    Erikson's Theory of Psychosocial Development
        Theoretical Framework
        Stages
        Nursing Application
    Piaget's Theory of Cognitive Development
        Theoretical Framework
        Stages
        Nursing Application
    Kohlberg's Theory of Moral Development
        Theoretical Framework
        Stages
        Nursing Application
    Social Learning Theory
        Theoretical Framework
        Nursing Application
    Behaviorism
        Theoretical Framework
        Nursing Application
    Ecologic Theory
        Theoretical Framework
        Nursing Application
    Temperament Theory
        Theoretical Framework
        Nursing Application
Influences on Development
    Genetics
    Prenatal Influences
    Other Influences
        Family Structure
        School
        Stress

        Socioeconomic Influences
        Community
        Culture
        Media
Infant (Birth- I Year)
    Physical Growth and Development
    Cognitive Development
    Play
    Nutrition
        Early Breast- or Bottle-Feeding
        Introduction of Other Foods
    Injury Prevention
    Personality and Temperament
    Communication
Toddler (1-3 Years)
    Physical Growth and Development
    Cognitive Development
    Play
    Nutrition
    Injury Prevention
    Personality and Temperament
    Communication
Preschool Child (3-6 Years)
    Physical Growth and Development
    Cognitive Development
    Play
    Nutrition
    Injury Prevention
    Personality and Temperament
    Communication
School-Age Child (6-12 Years)
    Physical Growth and Development
    Cognitive Development
    Play
    Nutrition
    Injury Prevention
    Personality and Temperament
    Communication
Adolescent (12-18 Years)
    Physical Growth and Development
    Cognitive Development
    Activities
    Nutrition
    Injury Prevention
    Personality and Temperament
    Communication
    Sexuality

Tables

Overhead Transparencies

Audio-Visual Resources

1. *Children's Drawings*
   Videocassette, 34 minutes
   Source: Health Sciences Consortium

2. *Interviewing Children: The Initial Assessment*
   Videocassette, 34 minutes
   Source: University of Michigan Media Library

3. *Everybody Rides the Carousel*
   16 mm, 72 minutes
   Source: University of Michigan Media Library

4. *The Infant*
   Videocassette, 38 minutes
   Source: American Journal of Nursing Co.

5. *Infant Development*
   Videocassette, 58 minutes
   Source: Johnson and Johnson

6. *Child Development: The First Two Years*
   Videocassette, 47 minutes
   Source: American Journal of Nursing Co.

7. *The Infant and Toddler Years*
   Videocassette, 21 minutes
   Source: Medcom/Trainex-Nasco Health Care Educational Materials

8. *The Toddler*
   Videocassette, 40 minutes
   Source: American Journal of Nursing Co.

9. *The Preschool Years*
   Videocassette, 17 minutes
   Source: Medcom/Trainex-Nasco Health Care Educational Materials

10. *The Preschool Child*
    Videocassette, 41 minutes
    Source: American Journal of Nursing Co.

11. *The School-Age Child*
    Videocassette, 41 minutes
    Source: American Journal of Nursing Co.

12. *The School Age Years*
    Videocassette, 16 minutes
    Source: Medcom/Trainex-Nasco Health Care Educational Materials

13. *The Pre-Adolescent Years*
    Videocassette, 19 minutes
    Source: Medcom/Trainex-Nasco Health Care Educational Materials
14. *Growing Up: Body, Feelings, and Behavior*
    Videocassette or 16 mm, 18 minutes
    Source: Churchill Films
15. *The Adolescent*
    Videocassette, 44 minutes
    Source: American Journal of Nursing Co.
16. *Adolescent Physical and Psychosocial Changes: Basis for Nursing Approaches*
    Videocassette, 30 minutes
    Source: Health Sciences Consortium

Potential Problem Areas for Students

1. Students may not accurately recall the laws of Mendelian inheritance. Overhead transparencies that depict dominant, recessive, and X-linked inheritance patterns would review and reinforce this information.
2. The stages of Piaget's theory of cognitive development are often difficult for students to remember. A chart that lists each stage, age of occurrence, and the most typical behaviors would condense and simplify this material.
3. Communicating with children of different ages may be difficult for students who have had little previous exposure to children. A review of cognitive and communication milestones may help students to relate appropriately to each age group.

Activities to Foster Critical Thinking

A. CLASSROOM ACTIVITIES

1. Utilize toy advertisements in magazines or toy catalogs as a basis for student critiques of toy safety and appropriateness for children of various ages.
2. Following presentation of influences on development, divide students into two groups to argue the relative contributions of hereditary and environmental factors.
3. Have students select the developmental theory that they consider the most applicable to nursing and defend their choice by developing nursing interventions for children in each developmental stage from that theory.
4. Show a recommended film for selected developmental stage. Ask students to identify specific nursing implications for caring for a child of that age from its content.

B. CLINICAL ACTIVITIES

1. Arrange for students to observe the activities of a child life specialist and describe the facets of development that are encouraged in each child.
2. Assign a developmental assessment to promote the formal evaluation of a child's developmental status.
3. Assign a process recording with a small child. Have the student critique the interchange.
4. Have students identify safety hazards in the clinical area.

3

PEDIATRIC ASSESSMENT

Chapter Overview

Chapter 3 presents the comprehensive assessment of children, encompassing both physical assessment and evaluation of developmental status. It assesses the unique anatomic and physiologic characteristics of children as well as techniques of history-taking and general appraisal. Most of the chapter discusses the components of a complete physical assessment, proceeding by body section or system. The final section correlates growth with nutritional status and presents a summary of developmental screening tests. Finally, the material that has been presented is applied to the opening case study to demonstrate the derivation of nursing actions from a comprehensive pediatric assessment.

Learning Objectives

- Obtain a thorough history, including patient information, physiologic data, and psychosocial data.
- Describe strategies to increase the cooperation of children during the physical examination.
- Select appropriate assessment techniques for each body system being examined.
- Describe normal and abnormal findings for each body system.
- Discuss the normal sequence of development found in boys and girls during puberty.
- Distinguish among the primitive reflexes found in infants.

Key Terms

assessment
auscultation
clinical judgement
effective communication
inspection
nonverbal behavior
palpation
percussion
range of motion
review of systems

Chapter Outline

Assessing the Heart for Heart Sounds and Function
Inspection of the Precordiurn
Palpation of the Precordium
Apical Impulse
Abnormal Sensations
Percussion of the Heart Borders
Auscultation of the Heart
Heart Rate and Rhythm
Differentiation of Heart Sounds
Splitting of the Heart Sounds
Third Heart Sound
Murmurs
Completing the Heart Examination
Blood Pressure
Palpation of the Pulses
Other Signs
Assessing the Abdomen for Shape, Bowel Sounds, and
Underlying Organs
Topographic Landmarks of the Abdomen
Inspection of the Abdomen
Shape
Umbilicus
Rectus Muscle
Abdominal Movement
Auscultation of the Abdomen
Percussion of the Abdomen
Palpation of the Abdomen
Light Palpation
Deep Palpation
Assessment of the Inguinal Area
Inspection
Palpation
Assessing the Genital and Perineal Areas for Pubertal
Development and External Structural Ab-
normalities
Preparation of Children for the Examination
Inspection of the Female Genitalia
Mons Pubis
Labia
Hymen
Urethral and Vaginal Openings
Vaginal Discharge
Palpation of Female Genitalia
Inspection of the Male Genitalia
Penis
Scrotum
Pubic Hair
Palpation of the Male Genitalia

Penis Testicles Spermatic Cord Enlarged Scro-
tum Cremasteric Reflex
Inspection of the Anus and Rectum Palpation of the
Anus and Rectum
Patency of the Anus Rectal Examination
Assessing the Musculoskeletal System for Bone and Joint
Structure, Movement, and Muscle Strength
Inspection of the Bones, Muscles, and Joints
Bones and Muscles
Joints
Palpation of the Bones, Muscles, and Joints
Bones and Muscles
Joints
Range of Motion and Muscle Strength Assessment
Active Range of Motion
Passive Range of Motion
Muscle Strength
Posture and Spinal Alignment
Posture
Spinal Alignment
Inspection of the Upper Extremities
Arms
Hands
Nails
Inspection of the Lower Extremities
Hips
Legs
Feet
Assessing the Nervous System for Cognitive Function,
Balance, Coordination, Cranial Nerve Func-
tion, Sensation, and Reflexes
Cognitive Function
Behavior
Communication Skills
Memory
Level of Consciousness
Cerebellar Function
Balance
Coordination
Gait
Cranial Nerve Function
Sensory Function
Superficial Tactile Sensation
Superficial Pain Sensation
Infant Primitive Reflexes
Superficial and Deep Tendon Reflexes
Superficial Reflexes
Deep Tendon Reflexes

Tables

Overhead Transparencies

Audio-Visual Resources

Source: American Journal of Nursing Co.
6. *Pediatric Anthropometry*
   Videocassette, 16 minutes
   Source: Rose Laboratories
7. *Physical Examination of the Preschool Child*
   Videocassette, 32 minutes
   Source: Career Aids
8. *Neurological Assessment of the Pediatric Patient*
   Videocassette, 28 minutes
   Source: American Journal of Nursing Co.
9. *SEARCH: The Art of Observation in Pediatrics*
   Videocassette, 16 minutes
   Source: Health Sciences Consortium

Potential Problem Areas for Students

1. Students may not be aware of the barriers to assessment that may be presented by children in different stages of development. Showing a film that demonstrates techniques of examining children of various ages may be helpful. A hand-out that outlines potential barriers by developmental age and lists techniques for overcoming these barriers could be used both as a guide for discussion of the film and a reference in the clinical area.
2. Infant primitive reflexes comprise a new area for Students and may be difficult to remember. The information presented in this chapter on the testing techniques of the principle reflexes and the timing of their appearance and extinction could be summarized on a hand-out for clinical reference and conference.

Activities to Foster Critical Thinking

A. CLASSROOM ACTIVITIES

1. Assign small groups of students to role-play the following data collection activities with a child and parent: history of present and past individual and family illnesses, review of systems, daily living patterns, and developmental data. Have class identify the principles demonstrated by the interviewer, cues provided by the child or parent, and actual or potential nursing diagnoses that could be derived from each interview.
2. Show a recommended audio-visual program that demonstrates the physical assessment of a child.

Have students discuss:
   (a) any problems the examiner encountered or might have encountered with each age group, infants, toddlers, preschoolers, school-age children, adolescents;
   (b) approaches for overcoming these problems with each age group; and
   (c) special communication techniques utilized by the examiner
3. Invite a pediatric dietitian to speak to the class about nutritional issues in the various developmental age groups. Following this presentation, have students answer the following questions:
   (a) What questions need to be asked to screen for nutritional status in each age group?
   (b) What physical signs would be significant in children with dietary deficiencies?
   (c) What cultural dietary practices might put children at risk for nutritional deficiencies?
4. Assign small groups of students to research the various developmental screening tests listed in Table 3-29. Have each group summarize the particular test and present it for class discussion.

B. CLINICAL ACTIVITIES

1. Assign students to perform an assessment of a child in the clinical area, analyze the data, and develop a plan of care for the child and family from this data.
2. Have each student observe a pediatrician or nurse practitioner conducting a comprehensive assessment in an ambulatory setting. At clinical conference, have each student present a critique of this activity for group discussion.
3. Require students to conduct a dietary screening that includes a 24-hour recall of food intake on their assigned patients. Have them analyze their findings and develop a teaching plan that:
   (a) overcomes any actual problems and
   (b) addresses the specific developmental issues of the age group.
4. Assign students to care for an infant in the clinical area and evaluate the primitive reflexes for normalcy.
5. Assign students to perform a selected developmental screening test and analyze the results.
6. Have students observe the developmental screening tests used in a variety of clinical settings and report on these in clinical conference for comparison.

4

Nursing Considerations for the Hospitalized Child

Chapter Overview

Chapter 4 presents a detailed description of the nurse's role in caring for ill children and their families in the hospital setting. It examines the effects of illness on both the child and family, discussing children's ability to comprehend illness by developmental age group. This information is used in the subsequent discussion of preparation for and adaptation to hospitalization. A variety of nursing strategies, including therapeutic play, are presented to assist the child and family with adaptation in a host of hospital situations. A discussion of issues related to long-term care, rehabilitation, and home care concludes this chapter.

Learning Objectives

- Describe children's understanding of health and illness from infancy through adolescence.
- Identify strategies to minimize separation anxiety in young children.
- Discuss strategies to decrease a child's fear of admission to the hospital.
- Discuss the stressors on the family when a child is admitted to the hospital.
- Describe the family's role in helping a child adapt to hospitalization.
- Identify strategies to promote coping and normal development during a child's hospitalization.
- Describe age-appropriate therapeutic play techniques.
- Describe how and when to prepare children for medical procedures.
- Outline a care plan for a child undergoing surgery.

Key Terms

case manager
child life specialist
individualized education plan
rehabilitation
rooming in
separation anxiety
therapeutic play

Chapter Outline

Effects of Illness and Hospitalization on Children and Families
    Children's Understanding of Health and Illness
        Infant
        Toddler and Preschooler
        School-Age Child
        Adolescent
    Family Responses to Hospitalization
Preparation for Hospitalization

Adaptation to Hospitalization
　　Special Units and Types of Care
　　　　Emergency Care
　　　　Intensive Care
　　　　Preoperative and Postoperative Areas
　　　　Short Stay Units
　　　　Isolation
　　　　Rehabilitation
　　Family Assessment
　　Child and Family Teaching
　　　　Teaching Plans
　　　　Children with Special Needs
　　Strategies to Promote Coping and Normal Development
　　　　Child Life Programs
　　　　Rooming in
　　　　Therapeutic Play
　　　　Therapeutic Recreation
　　Strategies to Meet Educational Needs
　　Preparation for Procedures
　　　　Preparation for Surgery
　　　　Preoperative Care
　　　　Postoperative Care
Preparation for Long-Term Care
Preparation for Home Care
　　Assessing the Child in Preparation for Discharge
　　Home Care Teaching
　　Preparing Parents to Act as Case Managers

Tables

Audio-Visual Resources

1. Communicating with Children: Supportive Interactions in Hospitals
   Videocassette with Study Guide, 120 minutes (6 segments)
   Source: Assoc. for the Care of Children's Health
2. *Preparing the Child for the Hospital Experience*
   Videocassette, 28 minutes
   Source: American Journal of Nursing Co.
3. A *Hospital Adventure: Starring Boris the Bear*
   Videocassette, 11 minutes
   Source: American Journal of Nursing Co.
4. *Promoting Normal Growth in the Hospitalized Child*
   Videocassette, 12 minutes
   Source: American Journal of Nursing Co.
5. *Young Children's Reaction to Hospitalization*
   Videocassette, 12 minutes
   Source: American Journal of Nursing Co.
6. *Initial Nursing Assessment of a Hospitalized Child Basis for Developing a Nursing Care Plan*
   Videocassette, 36 minutes
   Source: Health Sciences Consortium
7. *Nursing Care of the Hospitalized Child with a Chronic Health Problem*
   Videocassette, 28 minutes
   Source: Health Sciences Consortium
8. *Discharge Planning in Pediatric Catastrophic Illness*
   Videocassette, 56 minutes (2 parts)
   Source: American Journal of Nursing Co.
9. *Caring for Sick Children*
   Videocassette, 28 minutes
   Source: Films for the Humanities and sciences
10. *Family-Centered Care*
    Videocassette or 16 mm film with Study Guide, 38 minutes (original version), or 25 minutes (short version) with *A Film Study Guide for Nurses* (34 pages) available separately
    Source: Association for the Care of Children's Health
11. *Seasons of Caring*
    Videocassette, 40 minutes
    Source: Association for the Care of Children's Health

Potential Problem Areas for Students

1. Students may not grasp the varying impact of hospitalization on children and their families according to the type of unit and illness situation. Providing a comprehensive tour of a children's hospital or showing a film about children in a hospital setting could make them aware of the range of experiences and their potential effects.

2. Therapeutic play is likely to be a new concept for students and may be difficult for them to incorporate in their care. Having a child life specialist speak to the group and provide a list of age-specific activities prior to their clinical experience could provide a better understarding and a practice base.

Activities to Foster Critical Thinking

A. CLASSROOM ACTIVITIES

1. Invite a child life specialist or an experienced pediatric nurse to speak to class about preparation of the child for hospitalization and therapeutic play techniques. Following the presentation, have students identify specific problems and strategies related to both areas for the various developmental age groups.

2. Present a case study of a preschool child requiring ventilator assistance who is being discharged to home care. Ask students to participate in child's discharge planning, addressing:
   (a) assessment for discharge,
   (b) parental teaching,
   (c) community support services, and
   (d) issues related to ongoing care.

3. Show one of the recommended films related to the hospitalization of a child. Have students write a two-page reaction paper that addresses the impact of hospitalization portrayed in the film and nursing strategies to minimize these effects on the child.

4. Have each student research and prepare an oral report on the stressors and nursing strategies for children and parents in one of the following:
   (a) the emergency room,
   (b) the intensive care unit,
   (c) day surgery,
   (d) post anesthesia recovery,
   (e) short stay units,
   (f) isolation rooms, or
   (g) rehabilitation units.
   When reports have been presented about all of these areas, initiate group discussion to identify the commonalities and differences.

B. CLINICAL ACTIVITIES

1. Assign students to work with a child life specialist for a day. At clinical conference, have students describe activities and observed outcomes in terms of the developmental age group and clinical situation.

2. Identify a child in the clinical area who has a specific need for preparation. Have students develop, implement, and evaluate a teaching plan to prepare the child and family for the specific procedure or event.

3. Require students to develop and implement appropriate strategies of therapeutic play for the age and situation of each child they care for in the clinical area.

4. Assign students to follow a child and family from admission for day surgery through discharge, and develop, implement, and evaluate a family-centered care plan.

5. Assign students to follow the discharge planning nurse and describe the various components of this role.

6. Assign students to care for a child with multisystem problems who is being prepared for discharge. Have them work with the child's primary nurse in preparing the family and child for the transition to home care or a long-term care facility.

5

Nursing Considerations for the Child in the Community

Chapter Overview

New to the second edition, Chapter 5 is devoted to the care of children in community settings, whether in the home, school, care center, or wherever else children may be cared for. The role of the nurse in caring for children, including health promotion, supervision, developmental and family assessment, as well as home health care and care of children with acute and chronic conditions.

Learning Objectives

* Describe the nurse's role in health supervision and health promotion for children.
* Discuss the health supervision recommendations for children in specific age groups.
* Discuss health promotion in the community for children with chronic illnesses.
* Describe the rationale for developmental screening.
* Discuss the uses of developmental screening tests.
* List factors in the community that can have a negative effect on a child's growth and development.
* Describe methods to assess a family for strengths, resilience, coping skills, and resources.
* Explain the focus of home care nursing for medically fragile children.

Key Terms

chronic condition
developmental surveillance
disability
health supervision
medical home
medically fragile
screening tests
sensitivity
specificity

Chapter Outline

Health Supervision
    Nursing Assessment
        Disease and Injury Prevention
        Developmental Surveillance
    Nursing Diagnoses
    Nursing Management
        Provide Anticipatory Guidance
        Encourage Health Promotion Activities
        Perform Health Supervision Interventions
    Health Supervision by Age Group
        Infancy (Birth to 1 Year)
        Early Childhood (1-5 Years)
        Middle Childhood (5-12 Years)

Adolescence (12-18 Years)
Health Promotion for Children in Community Settings
    Episodic Care for Illnesses and Injuries
    Care of the Child With Special Health Care Needs
    Nursing in a School Setting
    Nurse's Role in Other Community Settings
Family Assessment
    Nursing Assessment
        Family Assessment Tools
        Home Assessment Tools
    Nursing Diagnoses
    Nursing Management
Home Health Care Nursing
    Nursing Assessment
        Transition from the Hospital
    Nursing Management

Tables

Overhead Transparencies

Audio-Visual Resources

1. *Children's Health in the Community*
   Videocassette, 40 minutes
   Source: Insight Media
2. *Raising Healthy Kids*
   Videocassette, 24 minutes
   Source: Films for the Humanities and Sciences
3. *Preventing Injuries to Children*
   Videocassette, 19 minutes
   Source: Films for the Humanities and Sciences
4. *Kids and Doctors*
   Videocassette, 19 minutes
   Source: Films for the Humanities and Sciences
5. *Competency in Childhood: Healthy Development*
   Videocassette, 24 minutes
   Source: J. B. Lippincott Company
6. *The Special Child: Maximizing Limited Potential*
   Videocassette, 26 minutes
   Source: Films for the Humanities and Sciences
7. *Family Assessment*
   Videocassette, 30 minutes
   Source: Insight Media
8. *Keeping the Balance*
   Videocassette, 23 minutes
   Source: Fanlight Productions
9. *Delivering Family-Centered, Home-Based Services*
   Videocassette, 52 minutes
   Source: Association for the Care of Children's Health

Potential Problem Areas for Students

1. Students are often unfamiliar with the roles and responsibilities of pediatric nurses in areas other than the acute care setting. Providing a summary of the concepts and goals identified in the *Standards and Guidelines for Pre-Licensure and Early Professional Education for Nursing Care of Children and Their Families*, available from the Society of Pediatric Nurses, could promote better understanding of the scope of pediatric nursing practice.

2. Students may have difficulty developing a plan of care for children and families in community settings. Providing sample nursing care plans that illustrate how each step of the nursing process is put into operation in various pediatric community settings could assist them in acquiring this competence.

Activities to Foster Critical Thinking

A. CLASSROOM ACTIVITIES

1. Assign students to investigate the role of the nurse in their choice of a pediatric community setting and report their findings to the class. Focus subsequent discussion to compare and contrast these roles.
2. Invite a nurse from a pediatric community setting to speak to the class about the specific nursing role, the population served, problems encountered, and nursing strategies employed. Have each student submit a written question for the speaker in advance.
3. Show one of the recommended audio-visual programs. Have the class discuss its implications for promoting the care of children and their families in the community.
4. Have students describe the activities of a school nurse from their own elementary, junior high, or high school. Focus discussion on whether these activities reflect the current Standards of School Nursing Care.
5. Present a case study of a child with a chronic illness who is receiving home care. Ask the students to discuss: (a) the impact of the situation on other family members, and (b) nursing interventions to lessen this impact.

B. CLINICAL ACTIVITIES

1. Arrange for students to spend a day in a pediatric clinic or pediatrician's office. Require them to identify:
   (a) methods utilized to assess children's growth and development,
   (b) specific health promotion activities,
   (c) anticipatory guidance provided, and
   (d) the role of the nurse in this setting.
2. Have students interview a nurse in a pediatric primary care clinic, pediatric specialty clinic, school, or home care organization. Have them determine:
   (a) the components of the nursing role,
   (b) preparation and previous nursing experience, and
   (c) specific skills required.
3. Assign students to follow a nurse in an early childhood education or school setting to observe direct care, teaching activities, and team planning meetings. Require them to develop a teaching plan that would be appropriate for that setting.
4. Assign students to work with a pediatric home health nurse and describe the various components of this role.
5. Have students interview the parent of a child with a chronic illness regarding the child's problem, daily care requirements, problems encountered, impact on family life, and community supports. Have them present this information in case study form.

6

The Child with a Life-Threatening Illness or Injury

Chapter Overview

Chapter 6 examines the experience of a life-threatening illness or injury in childhood from the perspective of the affected child, the parents, the siblings, and the nurse. In dealing with the child's perspective, it presents both stressors and coping mechanisms to be considered. Potential parental and sibling reactions to both a life-threatening situation and the death of the child are described in detail. Nursing management of both situations is fully discussed and applied in the form of a nursing care plan designed for a child coping with a life-threatening illness or injury. The chapter concludes with an examination of staff reactions following the death of a child on the unit.

Learning Objectives

- Describe the stressors of hospitalization for children in various developmental stages.
- Discuss nursing measures that will minimize the stressors of hospitalization in children.
- Identify the five stages of parental reaction when a child becomes critically ill or injured.
- Describe the needs of parents during the hospitalization of their critically ill child.
- Describe the reaction of siblings to the illness of a brother or sister.
- Identify nursing strategies for working with siblings of a critically ill child.

- Discuss parents' reactions to the death of their child.
- Discuss siblings' reactions to the death of a brother or sister.
- Describe children's understanding of and reaction to death according to their age group.
- Examine your own responses to death and dying.

Key Terms

death anxiety
death imagery
family crisis
hospice
stranger anxiety
support systems

Chapter Outline

Life-Threatening Illness or Injury
Child's Experience
    Stressors to the Child
        Infant
        Toddler
        Preschooler
        School-Age Child
        Adolescent
    Coping Mechanisms
    Nursing Assessment
    Nursing Diagnosis
    Nursing Management

Tables

Audio-Visual Resources

1. *Red Flags in the Critically Unstable Pediatric Patient*
   Videocassette with Study Guide, 28 minutes
   Source: American Journal of Nursing Co.
2. *The ABCs of Pediatric Trauma Nursing*
   Videocassette with Study Guide, 28 minutes
   Source: American Journal of Nursing Co.
3. *Emergency Assessment of the Traumatized Child*
   16 mm, 46 minutes
   Source: Medical Electronic Education Services
4. *Parenting in Pediatric Intensive Care*
   Videocassette, 16 minutes
   Source: Association for the Care of Children's Health
5. *When Children Grieve*
   Videocassette, 20 minutes
   Source: Churchill Films
6. *Where Is Dead?*
   16 mm, 19 minutes
   Source: Encyclopedia Britannica Corporation
7. *Jeannie*
   Videocassette, 6 minutes
   Source: Health Sciences Consortium
8. *Julie and John*
   Videocassette, 35 minutes
   Source: Health Sciences Consortium
9. *To Touch Today*
   Videocassette, 24 minutes
   Source: Health Sciences Consortium
10. *Letting Go*
    Videocassette, 29 minutes
    Source: American Journal of Nursing Co.

Potential Problem Areas for Students

1. Students caring for a child with a critical illness or injury may be overwhelmed by the challenges of providing complex physical care. Further, they may be emotionally overwhelmed by the situation and unable to respond to the supportive needs of the child and parents. Showing a recommended film and discussing the issues raised before their clinical experience allows students to examine their own feelings. It will help educate them to the complex needs of the child and family and prepare them to deal more adequately with a child's life-threatening situation.

Activities to Foster Critical Thinking

A. CLASSROOM ACTIVITIES

1. Assign students to submit a two-page paper describing a personal experience they have had with the critical illness or death of a family member or friend. Quote anonymous excerpts in class to illustrate common feelings, coping mechanisms, and examples of support or negative incidents during the experience. Ask the class to suggest ways nurses might provide support in the situations discussed.

2. Show one of the recommended films. Ask students to write down:
   (a) their major concern if they were assigned to care for this child,
   (b) one nursing intervention for the child, and
   (c) one nursing intervention for the family. List key points on overhead transparencies, and use as a basis for class discussion.

3. Invite a PICU nurse, a children's emergency room nurse, or a pediatric clinical nurse specialist to speak to the class about caring for children with life-threatening conditions. Have each student submit a written question in advance for the speaker.

4. Present a case study of a school-age child admitted to the PICU in a coma following a car accident from which both parents and a preschool-age sibling escaped without injury. Ask students to identify possible reactions of the family members and reasons for these behaviors.

5. Ask students to recall their concept of death when they were children. List responses on a transparency and have students determine the developmental stage each response reflects.

B. CLINICAL ACTIVITIES

1. Arrange for students to spend a day in an emergency room or PICU and observe the role of the nurse in caring for children with critical conditions and their families. Have students share their observations at clinical conference as a basis for discussion.

2. Assign students to care for a child with a life-threatening condition and develop an individualized nursing care plan for the child and family. Have them use the care plan to focus their discussion of the experience in clinical conference.

3. Have students interview a nurse who works in a critical care area regarding personal reactions to:
   (a) caring for children with life-threatening conditions,
   (b) caring for dying children, and
   (c) caring for parents and other family members in these situations.

4. Have students survey the physical arrangement of a pediatric critical care unit or emergency room and identify:
   (a) provisions for privacy,
   (b) provisions for parental comfort, and
   (c) the presence of helpful literature or lists for families.

PAIN ASSESSMENT AND MANAGEMENT

Chapter Overview

Chapter 7 provides an in-depth description of the assessment and management of pain from a developmental perspective. It addresses the physiologic basis of pain and its consequences before presenting useful behavioral indicators of pain and assessment scales for children. Discussion of pain management focuses on the opioids, NSAIDs, methods of analgesic administration, and nonpharmacological approaches to pain control in children. A narrative discussion of the nursing management of pain, a nursing care plan for a child with postoperative pain synthesizes and applies the chapter content to practice.

Learning Objectives

- Discuss cultural influences on pain in children.
- Explore the effect of the caregiver's cultural background in caring for children in pain.
- Describe physiologic responses and consequences of pain.
- Discuss the types of pain assessment scales.
- Describe the differences in children's understanding of and response to pain according to developmental stage.
- Describe the use of selected pain assessment scales.
- Differentiate between the side effects of narcotic and nonnarcotic analgesics.
- Discuss the use of patient-controlled analgesia

(PCA) in children.
- Describe various nonpharmacologic interventions to control pain in children.
- Describe how to prepare children for painful procedures.

Key Terms

acute
pain
anxiolysis
chronic pain
conscious sedation
deep sedation
distraction
electroanalgesia
equianalgesic dose
NSAIDs
opioids
pain
patient-controlled analgesia
tolerance

Chapter Outline

Outdated Beliefs about Pain in Children
Pain Indicators
    Physiologic Indicators
    Behavioral Indicators
    Consequences of Pain

Pain Assessment
    Pain History
    Cultural Influences on Pain
    Pain Assessment Scales
Medical Management of Pain
    Opioids
    Nonsteroidal Antiinflammatory Drugs
    Drug Administration
Nursing Management of Pain
    Increase and Maintenance of Patient Comfort
        Pharmacologic Intervention
        Nonpharmacologic Intervention
    Discharge Planning and Home Care Teaching
Pain Associated with Medical Procedures
    Medical Management
    Nursing Management
Increase Comfort During Painful Procedures

Tables

Overhead Transparencies

Audio-Visual Resources

1. *No Fears, No Tears*
   Videocassette, 27 minutes
   Source: Association for the Care of Children's Health
2. *Why Do I Have to Cry? Assessment of Pain in Children*
   Videocassette, 25 minutes
   Source: American Journal of Nursing Co.
3. *Medicating Children*
   Videocassette, 23 minutes
   Source: American Journal of Nursing Co.
4. *Special Issues in Pain Control: Pediatric Plan*
   Videocassette, 19 minutes
   Source: Health Sciences Consortium
5. *Special Pain Problems: Pediatric and Elderly Patients*
   Videocassette, 28 minutes
   Source: American Journal of Nursing Co.

Potential Problem Areas for Students

1. Students may hold preconceived ideas about children's pain because of popular myths of their own cultural background. Raising these issues for discussion prior to presenting formal materials on pain assessment and management in children could enhance student understanding.

2. Students may not be able to relate pain indicators and appropriate pain management to each developmental stage. A hand out that lists indicators of pain, comprehension of pain, and management approaches by developmental stage could be used as both a classroom teaching tool and a clinical reference.

3. Calculation of recommended pediatric analgesic medication dosages may be a problem for students. A worksheet of sample problems requiring the use of the body weight method of calculating dosages would provide practice in this area.

Activities to Foster Critical Thinking

A. CLASSROOM ACTIVITIES

1. Present a case study of a child who is experiencing pain following a traumatic injury. Ask students to

identify the perceptions, manifestations, assessment scale, and management specific to this child's age and situation.

2. Show a recommended film on pediatric pain. Ask each student to write down one way in which the material was different from previously held beliefs about pain in children. Collect and utilize these responses as the basis of group discussion.

3. Present a series of overhead transparencies that illustrate the commonly-used pain assessment scales. Ask students to choose a correct scale for each childhood age group. Require that each choice be related to a developmental rationale.

4. Make the statement, "Patientcontrolled analgesia can be effectively used in children as young as four years of age." Divide the class into two groups, one to defend and one to argue against this position.

B. CLINICAL ACTIVITIES

1. Assign students to review patient records on the unit to determine methods of pain management and ask the assigned nurse to evaluate the effectiveness of the method for the particular child. Compare and contrast the findings in clinical conference.

2. Require students to conduct age appropriate pain assessments on children assigned to them who are at risk for experiencing pain. Ask them to identify any existing barriers to effective pain management in these children.

3. At clinical conference, ask students who have cared for a child in pain to compare the experience to their previous care of an adult experiencing pain. Focus the discussion on objective and subjective indicators of pain and pain relief, management method used, route of administration of analgesic agents, environmental factors, and short term management outcomes.

4. Assign students to spend a morning observing the techniques of pain management in children in the following areas: pediatric intensive care unit, pediatric emergency room, postanesthesia. recovery room, and ambulatory surgery unit. Have them present and compare their observations at clinical conference.

5. Have students interview a pediatric nurse to determine personal feelings about the following:
   (a) performing painful procedures on children,
   (b) caring for children with pain, and
   (c) dealing with parents whose child is experiencing pain.

8

ALTERATIONS IN FLUID, ELECTROLYTE, AND ACID–BASE BALANCE

Chapter Overview

Chapter 8 explores the implications of fluid, electrolyte, and acid-base balance for children and adolescents. Since infants and children react more quickly to imbalances than adults, this chapter explains the anatomic and physiologic differences between children and adults. Homeostasis of fluids and electrolytes, as well as the results of imbalances of sodium, potassium, calcium, and magnesium are discussed in detail. Acid-base imbalances, including respiratory and metabolic acidosis and alkalosis are included, along with nursing implications and management.

Learning Objectives

- Describe actions that place infants and children at risk for fluid and electrolyte imbalances.
- Describe the clinical assessment of fluid imbalances in children.
- Identify manifestations and treatment of clinical dehydration.
- Identify manifestations and treatment of edema.
- Describe the clinical assessment of electrolyte imbalances in children.
- Discuss the medical and nursing management of children with electrolyte imbalances.
- Identify foods and substances that are high in potassium, calcium, and magnesium.
- Discuss the normal mechanisms for maintaining acid–base balance in the body.

- Describe the role of the lungs and kidneys in acid–base balance.
- Compare and contrast the four types of acid–base imbalances.
- Interpret ABG results in a pediatric patient.
- Outline potential causes of each type of imbalance.
- Describe clinical manifestations and medical and nursing management of each imbalance.

Key Terms

acidemia
acidosis
alkalemia
alkalosis
body fluid
buffer
dehydration
electrolytes
extracellular fluid
filtration
hypertonic fluid
hypotonic fluid
interstitial fluid
intracellular fluid
intravascular fluid
isotonic fluid
oncotic pressure
osmolality osmosis
pH
saline

Chapter Outline

Anatomy and Physiology of Pediatric Differences
Fluid Volume Imbalances
    Extracellular Fluid Volume Imbalances
        Extracellular Fluid Volume Deficit (Dehydration)
        Extracellular Fluid Volume Excess
    Interstitial Fluid Volume Excess (Edema)
Electrolyte Imbalances
    Sodium Imbalances
        Hypernatremia
        Hyponatremia
    Potassium Imbalances
        Hyperkalemia
        Hypokalemia
    Calcium Imbalances
        Hypercalcemia
        Hypocalcemia
    Magnesium Imbalances
        Hypermagnesemia
        Hypomagnesemia
Clinical Assessment of Fluid and Electrolyte Imbalance
Physiology of Acid–Base Balance
    Buffers
    Role of the Lungs
    Role of the Kidneys
    Role of the Liver
Acid–Base Imbalances
    Respiratory Acidosis
    Respiratory Alkalosis
    Metabolic Acidosis
    Metabolic Alkalosis
    Mixed Acid–Base Imbalances

Tables

8-1   Electrolyte Concentration in Body Fluid Compartments
8-2   Health Conditions Contributing to Fluid Imbalance
8-3   Severity of Clinical Dehydration
8-4   Clinical Manifestations of Extracellular Fluid Volume Deficit
8-5   Oral Rehydration and Maintenance Fluids for Mild and Moderate Dehydration
8-6   Oral Rehydration Therapy Guidelines
8-7   Calculation of Intravenous Fluid Needs

8-8   Clinical Conditions that Cause Edema
8-9   Causes of Hypernatremia
8-10   Causes of Hyponatremia
8-11   Nursing Interventions for a Child Who has a Fluid Restriction
8-12   Risk Factor Assessment for Fluid Imbalances
8-13   Risk Factor Assessment for Electrolyte Imbalances
8-14   Summary of Clinical Assessment of Fluid Imbalances
8-15   Summary of Clinical Assessment of Electrolyte Imbalances
8-16   Important Buffers
8-17   How to Interpret Arterial Blood Gas Measurements
8-18   Causes of Respiratory Acidosis
8-19   Laboratory Values in Uncompensated and Compensated Respiratory Acidosis
8-20   Causes of Hyperventilation
8-21   Laboratory Values in Uncompensated and Compensated Respiratory Alkalosis
8-22   Techniques for Reducing Anxiety in Children With Parethesias
8-23   Causes of Metabolic Acidosis
8-24   Laboratory Values in Uncompensated and Compensated Metabolic Acidosis
8-25   Laboratory Values in Uncompensated and Compensated Metabolic Alkalosis
8-26   Causes of Metabolic Alkalosis

Overhead Transparency

Fig. 8-18   (A) Recycling of bicarbonate by the kidneys
Fig. 8-18   (B) Secretion and buffering of hydrogen ions in the kidneys

Audio-Visual Resources

1. *Pediatric IV Therapy*
   Videocassette, 40 minutes
   Source: American Journal of Nursing Co.
2. *Intravenous Therapy, Part I: Fluid and Electrolyte Balance*
   Videocassette, 28 minutes
   Source: Fairview General Hospital
3. *Fluid Balance: Assessment, Maintenance, Intervention*

Videocassette, 22 minutes
Source: Medcom/Trainex, Inc.

4. *Pediatric Physical Care: Fluid Balance and IV Therapy*
Slide-tape, 16 minutes
Source: Concept Media

5. *Assessing Fluids and Electrolytes*
Videocassette, 30 minutes
Source: Insight Media

6. *The Critical Balance, Part I*
Videocassette, 15 minutes
Source: Concept Media

7. *The Critical Balance, Part II*
Videocassette, 17 minutes
Source: Concept Media

8. *Potassium Balance*
Videocassette, 29 minutes
Source: Insight Media

9. *Maintenance and Compensation Balance*
Videocassette, 18 minutes
Source: Insight Media

10. *Ups and Downs of pH*
Videocassette, 16 minutes
Source: Concept Media

11. *Fluid and Electrolytes: Clinical Assessments and Interventions; Program 3: Acid-Base Balance*
Videocassette, 15 minutes
Source: J. B. Lippincott Company

12. *Respiratory Alkalosis and Acidosis*
Videocassette, 27 minutes
Source: Concept Media

13. *Metabolic Alkalosis and Acidosis*
Videocassette, 29 minutes
Source: Concept Media

Potential Problem Areas for Students

1. Students may not understand the age-associated differences in body fluid proportions and compartmental distribution. An overhead transparency that lists this information in chart form from infancy through adulthood would provide visual reinforcement when this material is presented.

2. It may be difficult for students to comprehend the physiological mechanisms underlying the various fluid imbalances. A chart that compares extracellular fluid volume imbalances and osmolality imbalances by definition, etiology, and clinical manifes-

tations could enhance clarity and promote understanding.

3. Students tend to try to memorize electrolyte imbalances without understanding their association with clinical manifestations. A hand-out in chart form that lists the principal imbalances with their major manifestations according to body system could assist with both classroom presentation and clinical application.

4. Students may not understand how the management of dehydration in infants and children is determined. Guidelines for rehydration, including type of fluid and rate of administration according to body weight and type and degree of dehydration, could serve as an explanation and clinical reference.

5. Students often do not understand the body's natural mechanisms for regulating acid-base balance, nor are they aware of regulatory differences in infants and young children. An overhead transparency that concisely presents the roles of the lungs, kidneys, and buffers in maintaining homeostasis and identifies pediatric variations could clarify these areas.

6. Students may not recognize arterial blood gas values that indicate a compensated acid-base imbalance. A hand-out chart that lists normal values and indicates the directional change of each value for each uncompensated and compensated imbalance could be helpful. This chart could be used initially in class to visually support the explanation of compensatory mechanisms and subsequently as a reference in the clinical area for evaluating children's blood gases.

7. Students may erroneously equate fully compensated imbalances with resolution. On the chart suggested above, include the following notation: Compensation reflects the effort of the regulatory mechanisms to return the pH to normal by making either the PCO_2 or HCO_3 abnormal. Resolution reflects correction of the underlying problem with return of all values to normal.

Activities to Foster Critical Thinking

A. CLASSROOM ACTIVITIES

1. Show the videotape, *"Fluid Balance: Assessment, Maintenance, Intervention."* Ask students to generate a list of assessment activities that they observed

for each type of fluid imbalance. Question them regarding the rationale for each of these activities.

2. Use overhead transparencies to present relevant laboratory values and clinical manifestations of the major electrolyte and acid-base imbalances. Display these in random order and ask students to:
   (a) identify the imbalance and
   (b) describe the nursing management of a child with this imbalance.

3. Present a case study of a young child with generalized edema. Ask students to identify:
   (a) possible causes,
   (b) strategies for monitoring the degree of edema,
   (c) relevant nursing diagnoses, and
   (d) nursing management activities.

4. Have students role-play a scenario in which a clinic nurse is instructing parents of an infant with moderate dehydration regarding management of the problem at home. Ask the remaining students to critique the instructions and the manner in which they were given.

5. Present a list of childhood illnesses that could produce acid-base imbalances. Have students identify:
   (a) the type of imbalance that might develop in each condition and
   (b) nursing assessment activities to identify and monitor that imbalance.

6. Present a case study of a toddler with severe croup who has developed uncompensated respiratory acidosis. Ask students to identify:
   (a) the underlying mechanisms for this imbalance,
   (b) the mechanism of compensation,
   (c) clinical manifestations and pertinent laboratory values,
   (d) nursing management strategies, and
   (e) the developmental issues to be considered in planning this child's care.

B. CLINICAL ACTIVITIES

1. Assign students to care for a child with a fluid, electrolyte, or acid-base imbalance. Have them evaluate the child's laboratory data and assess the child's hydration status before developing a nursing care plan.

2. At clinical conference, have each student present the pertinent IV information on the patient cared for. Ask students to analyze the types of fluid and rates of administration in relation to the child's condition and body weight.

3. Have students develop, implement, and evaluate a discharge teaching plan for parents who are taking a child home following hospitalization for a fluid, electrolyte, or acid-base imbalance.

4. Have students interview a nurse with experience in IV therapy to identify:
   (a) problems commonly encountered in establishing and maintaining a peripheral IV in children and
   (b) techniques for overcoming these problems.

5. Arrange for students to work with a dietitian who provides discharge teaching for a child and family regarding dietary prevention of future fluid, electrolyte, and acid-base imbalances. Discuss any problems encountered and strategies for dealing with these problems.

6. Arrange for child life specialist to speak at clinical conference to describe appropriate psychosocial support and therapeutic play activities for children on the unit who are receiving IV therapy.

7. Have students review the records of all children on the unit to determine the number and type of fluid, electrolyte, and acid-base imbalances currently being treated. Discuss findings in clinical conference.

8. Have students who have cared for both children and adults with fluid, electrolyte, or acid-base imbalances compare and contrast these experiences.

9

ALTERATIONS IN IMMUNE FUNCTION

Chapter Overview

Chapter 9 addresses the group of conditions related to altered immune function in children. A discussion of the physiology of the immune system that includes pediatric variations provides a theoretical base. Specific conditions are grouped as immunodeficiency disorders, autoimmune diseases, and allergic reactions. A nursing care plan for the child with AIDS applies the information to practice in a currently relevant pediatric condition that is also the subject of the chapter's introductory case study.

Learning Objectives

- Explain the normal immune response in children.
- Differentiate between B cell and T cell disorders.
- Describe the clinical manifestations and pathophysiology of immunodeficiency disorders.
- Describe the precautions used in caring for children with immunodeficiency disorders.
- Outline the nursing management of children with immunodeficiency disorders.
- Describe the clinical manifestations and pathophysiology of autoimmune disorders.
- Discuss the nursing management of children with selected autoimmune disorders.
- Outline the nursing mangement of children exhibiting hypersensitivity reactions.

Key Terms

allergen
antibody
antigen
graft-versus-host disease
hypersensitivity response
immunodeficiency
immunoglobulin
opportunistic infection
primary immune response

Chapter Outline

Tables

Overhead Transparency

Audio-Visual Resources

1. *Body Defenses against Disease*
   Videocassette or 16 mm, 14 minutes
   Source: Encyclopedia Britannica
2. *Care of HIV Infected Children*
   Videocassette with Study Guide, 28 minutes
   Source: American Journal of Nursing Co.
3. *Pediatric AIDS: A Time of Crisis*
   Videocassette or 16 mm, 23 minutes
   Source: Association for the Care of Children's Health
4. *AIDS: An Enemy Among Us*
   Videocassette, 45 minutes
   Source: Churchill Films
5. *AIDS, HIV and Seroconversion: What You Should Know*
   Videocassette with Study Guide, 20 minutes
   Source: Guidance Associates
6. *AIDS: Prevention for Nursing Professionals*
   Videocassette, 20 minutes
   Source: Guidance Associates
7. *A Letter from Brian*
   Videocassette, 29 minutes
   Source: American Red Cross, Los Angeles Chapter
8. *Living with Chronic Illness (JRA and SLE)*
   Videocassette, 33 minutes
   Source: Health Sciences Consortium
9. *Systemic Lupus Erythematosus—It Means Some Changes*
   Videocassette, 26 minutes
   Source: University of Michigan
10. *Allergies: The Twentieth Century Disease*
    Videocassette, 42 minutes
    Source: Filmmakers Library

Potential Problem Areas for Students

1. Students may neither recall the mechanisms of acquired immunity nor be aware of immune system differences in young children. An overhead transparency that presents acquired immunity in its parallel humoral and cellular components and highlights pediatric variations could deliver this material effectively.

2. Students may have difficulty understanding the differences among the various immunodeficiency diseases. An overhead transparency that lists each condition with its significant cellular or other immunological deficits could help with this differentiation.

Activities to Foster Critical Thinking

A. CLASSROOM ACTIVITIES

1. Show one of the recommended audio-visual programs about AIDS. Have students discuss issues it raises:
   (a) responsibility for transmission to children,
   (b) risks for nurses caring for children with AIDS,
   (c) quality of life in children with AIDS, and
   (d) societal attitudes.
2. Arrange for a nurse who works with the pediatric AIDS population to speak to the class about the experience and issues it raises for nurses. Have each student submit one written question for the speaker in advance.
3. Present a case study of a school-age child with juvenile rheumatoid arthritis or systemic lupus erythematosus. Have students identify:
   (a) issues related to development in a child with this condition and
   (b) nursing approaches to support normal development in this child.
4. Ask students with allergic conditions to identify themselves and share their experiences related to diagnosis, management, and education in which a nurse was involved. Have class evaluate nursing actions and suggest additional or modified approaches.

B. CLINICAL ACTIVITIES

1. Assign students to care for a child with AIDS, juvenile rheumatoid arthritis, or systemic lupus erythematosus and develop a comprehensive care plan for this child and family.
2. Have students interview nurses who have cared for young children with AIDS regarding their feelings and concerns. Have them inquire about support services that are available for staff in this facility working with these children.
3. Have students develop, implement, and evaluate a teaching plan for a child who is being discharged on long-term steroid therapy.
4. Have students to observe a physical therapist working with a child with juvenile rheumatoid arthritis. Have them report on techniques observed and the child's response to therapy. Ask them to identify ways nurses can support goals of physical therapy with these children.
5. Have students keep a list of the professionals who are observed providing care for a child with AIDS, juvenile rheumatoid arthritis, or systemic lupus erythematosus. Have them describe the role of each professional and evaluate whether their combined efforts result in holistic care for the child and family.
6. Have students follow a child life specialist working with children with AIDS or an autoimmune disorder and report what measures they observed that promoted normal development in these children.

10

INFECTIOUS AND COMMUNICABLE DISEASES

Chapter Overview

Chapter 10 discusses infectious and communicable diseases in children and adolescents. The process of infection and the special vulnerability of children are discussed, and immunizations are covered in detail. An extensive table covers 19 infectious and communicable diseases including a description of the problem, clinical manifestations, treatment, and nursing management.

Learning Objectives

- Discuss the chain of infection.
- Describe the factors that make children particularly vulnerable to infectious diseases.
- Differentiate between active and passive immunization and give examples of each.
- Outline the recommended schedule of vaccinations for all children.
- Describe the actions and documentation that are mandated when immunizations are given.
- Discuss the side effects, contraindications, and nursing considerations for pediatric immunizations.
- Describe immunization side effects that must be reported.
- Describe the mechanism of body temperature control.

- Describe a positive benefit of fever.
- Discuss the characteristics, clinical manifestations, treatment, and nursing management of selected infectious and communicable diseases in children.

Key Terms

acellular vaccine
active immunity
communicable diseases
direct transmission
indirect transmission
infectious disease
killed virus vaccine
live virus vaccine
nosocomial infection
passive immunity
toxoid
transplacental immunity

Chapter Outline

Special Vulnerability of Children
Immunization
    Nursing Assessment
    Nursing Diagnosis
    Nursing Management
Infectious and Communicable Diseases in Children

Clinical Manifestations
    Physiology of Fever
Diagnostic Tests and Medical Management
Nursing Assessment
Nursing Diagnosis
Nursing Management
    Care of the Child at Home
    Care of the Child in the Health Care Setting

Tables

Audio-Visual Resources

1. *Chain of Infection*
   Videocassette, 29 minutes
   Source: Concept Media
2. *How Infection Strikes*
   Videocassette, 20 minutes
   Source: Films for the Humanities and Sciences
3. *Bacteria and Viruses*
   Videocassette, 20 minutes
   Source: Films for the Humanities and Sciences
4. *Immunizations*
   Videocassette, 20 minutes
   Source: Films for the Humanities and Sciences
5. *Childhood Vaccines*
   Videocassette, 22 minutes
   Source: Films for the Humanities and Sciences
6. *Chicken Pox: Vaccinate and Prevent*
   Videocassette, 22 minutes
   Source: Films for the Humanities and Sciences
7. *Common Childhood Illnesses*
   Videocassette, 45 minutes
   Source: Films for the Humanities and Sciences
8. *Lyme Disease in Our Own Backyard*
   Videocassette, 56 minutes
   Source: Films for the Humanities and Sciences
9. *Whooping Cough*
   Videocassette, 21 minutes
   Source: Films for the Humanities and Sciences
10. *Respiratory Syncytial Virus: A Seasonal Dilemma*
    Videocassette, 16 minutes
    Source: J. B. Lippincott Company
11. *Nosocomial Pneumonia: Stopping It at the Source*
    Videocassette, 20 minutes
    Source: J. B. Lippincott Company
12. *Pediatric Antibiotic Resistance*
    Videocassette, 17 minutes
    Source: Films for the Humanities and Sciences
13. *Infection Control, Volumes 1 and 2*
    Two Videocassettes, 30 minutes each
    Source: Insight Media
14. *Basic Infection Control Measures*
    Videocassette, 25 minutes
    Source: Concept Media

Potential Problem Area for Students

1. Students may not be aware of the mechanisms of direct and indirect transmission of infection. Using an overhead transparency depicting the chain of infection to illustrate how transmission occurs may clarify this information.
2. Changing childhood immunization recommendations make it difficult for students to evaluate the immunization status of children. Distributing a copy of the current Recommended Childhood Immunization Schedule, United States, as a clinical hand-out would provide an accurate reference.
3. Students may not be aware of the potential adverse effects and contraindications associated with childhood immunizations. A hand-out that summarizes these entities would convey the necessary information and be available as a clinical reference.

Activities to Foster Critical Thinking

A. CLASSROOM ACTIVITIES

1. Invite a pediatric nurse from a clinic or pediatrician's office to speak to the class about childhood immunizations and infectious diseases. Focus class discussion around issues related to parent education, provisions for catch-up vaccinations, potential

contraindications, supplemental immunizations, and prevalence of specific infectious diseases in your area.

2. Following the presentation of material about the potential for serious adverse reactions to childhood immunizations, divide students into two groups for discussion. Have one group take the position that all immunizations must be given unless specifically contraindicated and the other argue against this on grounds of freedom of choice and safety.

3. Present a series of vignettes of the following childhood illnesses: chicken pox, coxsackievirus, fifth disease, measles, mumps, Lyme disease, rubella and streptococcal pharyngitis. For each disease, ask students to identify:
   (a) the causative organism,
   (b) any preventive measures available,
   (c) common clinical manifestations,
   (d) treatment measures and
   (e) prognosis.
   Have each student select one vignette and develop a nursing care plan for a child infected with that disease.

4. Assign students investigate issues related to pediatric antibiotic resistance and report their findings to the class.

5. Have students role-play a nurse responding to the following situations:
   (a) a 3-year-old child with no record of immunizations,
   (b) a parent who refuses to sign the consent form for the child's immunization,
   (c) a child whose immunization sequence has been interrupted, and
   (d) the unexpected arrival of a child with an infectious disease in a crowded clinic area.
   Ask the remaining students to critique the responses.

B. CLINICAL ACTIVITIES

1. Arrange for students to spend a day in a pediatric clinic or office and evaluate the immunization status of children that are seen.

2. Have students interview a nurse in a pediatric clinic or office to determine the prevalence of adverse events related to immunizations and the protocols that are followed as protection against professional liability.

3. Assign students to care for a child with an infectious disease in an acute care setting and develop an appropriate plan of care.

4. Arrange for students to follow an infection control nurse and identify:
   (a) the components of this role,
   (b) specific problems posed by childhood infections, and
   (c) strategies for dealing with these problems.

5. Have students develop, implement, and evaluate a family teaching plan for the home care of a child with an infectious disease.

11

ALTERATIONS IN
RESPIRATORY FUNCTION

Chapter Overview

Chapter 11 deals with both acute and chronic respiratory conditions in children. It discusses the upper and lower airway differences in adults and children and relates these variations to the assessment of commonly occurring pediatric respiratory disorders. These disorders are grouped for discussion as urgent respiratory threats, reactive airway disorders, lower airway disorders, and injuries of the respiratory system. A nursing care plan for the child with laryngotracheobronchitis applies the principles of nursing management of children with respiratory disorders to the management of a specific condition.

Learning Objectives

*   Explain the significance of the differences between adult and pediatric respiratory tracts.
*   Differentiate between early and late symptoms of respiratory distress.
*   Describe the nursing assessments performed on children in respiratory distress.
*   Describe the needs of the family of an infant who has died of sudden infant death syndrome (SIDS).
*   Differentiate among the types of reactive airway disorders.
*   Explain the nursing management of children with

acute and chronic respiratory disorders.
*   Discuss the medications frequently used to manage acute and chronic respiratory disorders.
*   Formulate discharge instructions for children with acute or chronic respiratory disorders.
*   Explain the multisystem changes that occur in children with cystic fibrosis.
*   Outline anticipatory guidance for parents of children who have unintentional injuries of the respiratory system.

Key Terms

adventitious
airway resistance
alveolar hypoventilation
apnea
dysphonia
dyspnea
hypercapnia
hypoxemia
hypoxia
laryngospasm
paradoxical breathing
periodic breathing
retractions
stridor
tachypnea
trigger

Chapter Outline

Anatomy and Physiology of Pediatric Differences
    Upper Airway Differences
    Lower Airway Differences
Urgent Respiratory Threats
    Apnea
        Apnea of Prematurity
        Apparent Life-threatening Event
        Nursing Management
    Sudden Infant Death Syndrome
        Nursing Management
    Respiratory Failure
        Nursing Management
Reactive Airway Disorders
    Croup Syndromes
        Laryngotracheobronchitis
        Epiglottitis (Supraglottitis)
        Bacterial Tracheitis
    Asthma
        Clinical Manifestations
        Etiology and Pathophysiology
        Diagnostic Tests and Medical Management
        Nursing Assessment
        Nursing Diagnosis
        Nursing Management
    Status Asthmaticus
Lower Airway Disorders
    Neonatal Respiratory Distress Syndrome
        Nursing Management
    Bronchopulmonary Dysplasia
        Nursing Management
    Bronchitis
        Nursing Management
    Bronchiolitis
        Clinical Manifestations
        Etiology and Pathophysiology
        Diagnostic Tests and Medical Management
        Nursing Assessment
        Nursing Diagnosis
        Nursing Management
    Pneumonia
        Nursing Management
    Tuberculosis
        Nursing Management
    Cystic Fibrosis
        Clinical Manifestations
        Etiology and Pathophysiology

Diagnostic Tests and Medical Management
    Nursing Assessment
    Nursing Diagnosis
    Nursing Management
Injuries of the Respiratory System
    Airway Obstruction
        Foreign Body Aspiration
    Near Drowning
        Nursing Management
    Smoke Inhalation Injury
        Nursing Management
    Blunt Chest Trauma
    Pulmonary Contusion
        Nursing Management
    Pneumothorax
        Nursing Management

Tables

11-18 Medications Used to Treat Bronchopulmonary Dysplasia
11-19 Medical Management of Bronchiolitis
11-20 Diagnostic Tests for Tuberculosis
11-21 Diagnostic Test for Cystic Fibrosis (Sweat Test)
11-22 Medical Management for Cystic Fibrosis

Overhead Transparency

Fig. 11-1 Respiratory anatomic and physiologic differences between children and adults (p. 409)

Audio-Visual Resources

1. *Acute Respiratory Distress in Children*
   Videocassette, 16 minutes
   Source: Network for Continuing Medical Education
   Roche Laboratories
2. *Management of Airway Obstruction*
   Videocassette, 11 minutes
   Source: Health Sciences Consortium
3. *Pediatric Physiotherapy*
   Videocassette, 10 minutes
   Source: Medical Electronic Educational Services, Inc.
4. *Suctioning Techniques for the Pediatric Patient*
   Videocassette, 10 minutes
   Source: Health Sciences Consortium
5. *Asthma*
   Videocassette, 52 minutes
   Source: Health Sciences Consortium
6. *A Regular Kid*
   16 min, 15 minutes
   Source: American Lung Association
7. *The Story of Sixty-Five Roses*
   16 mm, 10 minutes
   Source: Cystic Fibrosis Foundation
8. *The Story of Susan McKellar*
   Videocassette or 16 mm, *20* minutes
   Source: Filmmakers Library
9. *Don't Cry for Me*
   16 min, 54 minutes
   Source: Umbrella Films

Potential Problem Areas for Students

1. Students may memorize the airway differences between adults and children without understanding their clinical significance. Overhead transparencies that provide parallel lists of each pediatric upper and lower airway difference with its accompanying significance could resolve this difficulty.
2. Students tend to think of croup as a single disorder, rather than a group of closely related upper airway conditions. Use of a chart that presents the types of croup by etiology, age, onset, manifestations, and severity could help to clarify and organize information about the croup syndromes for presentation.
3. Students often memorize nursing management strategies for each specific respiratory disorder instead of linking nursing actions to their underlying rationales. A hand-out that presents these nursing actions in the categories of assessment, pharmacologic approaches, and nonpharmacologic approaches for each could be provided. This could promote understanding and allow for generalization of many management strategies to groups of respiratory disorders.

Activities to Foster Critical Thinking

A. CLASSROOM ACTIVITIES

1. Present a case study of an infant who has been hospitalized following an apneic episode. Have students identify factors to be considered when providing support to the parents. Ask them to discuss the following:
   (a) potential causes,
   (b) diagnostic protocols,
   (c) nursing management, and
   (d) elements of a parent teaching plan.
2. Arrange for a student to attend a SIDS support group meeting and report on this visit to the class. Have students discuss the immediate and long-term support that should be provided for the parents. Ask how the loss of a child to SIDS may affect the parenting of future children in that family.
3. Present a case study of a school-age child with asthma. Ask students to:
   (a) identify the potential psychosocial consequences of asthma in this age group and
   (b) discuss nursing management strategies to minimize these problems.
4. Present current incidence statistics for tuberculosis in the United States. Ask students what factors may

have contributed to its increased occurrence in your region.

5. Show a recommended film about cystic fibrosis. Have students discuss the quality of life issues it raises.

B. CLINICAL ACTIVITIES

1. Have students auscultate breath sounds on:
   (a) a peer,
   (b) an infant or young child with normal respiratory status, and
   (c) an infant or young child with a respiratory disorder.

Ask them to compare and contrast their findings and give reasons for the differences identified.

2. Assign students to care for a young child with a respiratory disorder and develop a comprehensive care plan for this child.

3. Arrange for students to follow a respiratory therapist who is delivering pediatric therapy. Have students observe assessment and treatment activities, evaluate their overall effectiveness, and describe how these activities differ from adult respiratory therapies.

4. Assign students to develop, implement and evaluate an age-appropriate teaching plan for a child hospitalized with a respiratory disorder.

12

ALTERATIONS IN CARDIOVASCULAR FUNCTION

Chapter Overview

Chapter 12 introduces both congenital and acquired disorders of cardiovascular function in children. The transition from fetal to pulmonary circulation and the subsequent pediatric differences in oxygenation and circulation are described. Specific conditions are presented, such as congestive heart failure, acquired heart disease, vascular diseases, and injuries to this system. A nursing care plan for a child with congestive heart failure synthesizes information presented in the opening case study, and nursing management issues that arise in many of the conditions are addressed.

Learning Objectives

- Compare the fetal and pulmonary circulation of the heart.
- Describe changes that occur in three fetal cardiovascular structures after birth.
- Discuss the child's response to chronic hypoxemia.
- Describe the etiology and clinical manifestations of congestive heart failure (CHF) and the medical and nursing management of children with this disorder.
- Differentiate between cyanotic and acyanotic heart defects.

- Discuss the anatomy and clinical manifestations of selected acyanotic heart defects and the medical and nursing management of children with these defects.
- Discuss the anatomy and clinical manifestations of cyanotic heart defects and the clinical and nursing management of children with these defects.
- Outline the diagnostic tests and procedures used to diagnose congenital heart diseases.
- Discuss the etiology of selected cardiac and vascular diseases and the medical and nursing management of children with these diseases.
- Discuss the etiology of selected injuries to the cardiovascular system and the medical and nursing management of children with these injuries.

Key Terms

compliance
desaturated blood
digitalization
hemodynamics
palliative procedure
polycythemia
preload
pulmonary hypertension
shunt
syncope

Chapter Outline

Anatomy and Physiology of Pediatric Differences
    Transition from Fetal to Pulmonary Circulation
        Oxygenation
        Cardiac Functioning
Congestive Heart Failure
        Clinical Manifestations
        Etiology and Pathophysiology
        Diagnostic Tests and Medical Management
        Nursing Assessment
        Nursing Diagnosis
        Nursing Management
Congenital Heart Disease
    Acyanotic Defects
        Nursing Care of the Child Undergoing a Cardiac Catheterization
        Nursing Care of the Child Undergoing Surgery for an Acyanotic Defect
    Cyanotic Defects
Acquired Heart Diseases
    Rheumatic Fever
        Nursing Management
    Infective Endocarditis
        Nursing Management
    Cardiac Arrhythmias
        Nursing Management
Vascular Diseases
    Kawasaki Disease
        Nursing Management
    Hyperlipidemia
        Nursing Management
    Hypertension
    Persistent Pulmonary Hypertension
Injuries of the Cardiovascular System
    Shock
        Hypovolemic Shock
        Distributive Shock
        Obstructive Shock
        Cardiogenic Shock
    Myocardial Contusion

Tables

Overhead Transparencies

Audio-Visual Resources

1. *Work of the Heart*
   Videocassette or 16 mm, 19 minutes
   Source: Encyclopedia Britannica Educational Corporation
2. *Your Baby with a Congenital Heart Defect*
   Videocassette, 29 minutes
   Source: University of Michigan
3. *Cardiac Failure in Infancy*
   16 mm, 30 minutes
   Source: American Heart Association
4. *Congenital Malformations of the Heart: Cyanotic Congenital Heart Disease*
   16 mm, 30 minutes
   Source: Universal Education and Visual Arts
5. *Congenital Malformations of the Heart: Acyanotic Congenital Heart Disease*
   16 mm, 14 minutes
   Source: Universal Education and Visual Arts
6. *Leonard Z Lion Presents: (a) Learning about Your Heart Catheterization; (b) Learning about Your Heart Operation;* (c) *Taking Care of Your Teeth to Protect Your Heart*
   Three videocassettes, 10-16 minutes
   Source: University of Michigan
7. *Jeannie*
   Videocassette, 6 minutes
   Source: Health Sciences Consortium

Potential Problem Areas for Students

1. Students may not recall the circulatory changes that normally occur at birth. An overhead transparency that presents a visual representation of the differences between fetal circulation and pulmonary circulation would review and clarify this material.
2. It may be difficult for students to distinguish between acyanotic and cyanotic heart defects. A handout that divides the common congenital heart defects into these categories and includes a diagram and description of each defect could assist with conceptualization.
3. Students may not be aware that blood volume differences in young children mandate early recogni-

tion of hypovolemic shock. An overhead transparency that presents blood volumes by age and weight and relates this information to clinical manifestations of shock in children could promote awareness of this issue.

Activities to Foster Critical Thinking

A. CLASSROOM ACTIVITIES

1. Show a recommended audio-visual program and have the class discuss the issues it raises. Ask students how the congenital heart defects may affect:
   (a) parent-child relationships and
   (b) the child's development.
2. Arrange for a nurse who cares for children with cardiac defects to speak to the class about the nurse's role at various stages of care. Have each student submit one question for the speaker in advance.
3. Present a series of situational vignettes related to children with acquired heart and vascular diseases. For each condition, have students identify:
   (a) appropriate nursing diagnoses,
   (b) nursing management strategies,
   (c) rationales to support these strategies, and
   (d) appropriate developmental considerations.
4. Invite a parent or professional involved in a support group for families of children with cardiac defects to speak to the class. Focus postpresentation discussion on the effects of the child's condition on the family and the nurse's supportive role in this area.

B. CLINICAL ACTIVITIES

1. Arrange for students to accompany a child for a cardiac catheterization. At clinical conference, have them report on the observed nurse's role and the reactions of the child to the experience.
2. Arrange for students to observe one of the following:
   (a) a child's cardiac surgery,
   (b) immediate postanesthesia recovery following cardiac surgery,
   (c) care of a child with a cardiac defect or following cardiac surgery in a PICU, or
   (d) postsurgical preparation for home care.

At clinical conference, compare and contrast these experiences in terms of nursing roles and the reactions of the child and family.

3. Assign students to care for a child with a congenital or acquired cardiac condition, vascular disease, or cardiovascular injury. Require that they develop a comprehensive care plan for the child and family.

4. Arrange for students to attend a support group meeting for families of children with cardiac defects. Have them note the issues raised related to the child, the parents, and the siblings and how support was provided.

5. Arrange for students to visit a children's cardiac clinic to observe children's experiences and the role of the nurse. Have them develop a case study from the visit to present for discussion at clinical conference.

Alterations in Hematologic Function

Chapter Overview

Chapter 13 focuses on the various childhood hematologic disorders. It examines hematologic differences in children, particularly related to red blood cells, white blood cells, and platelets. Specific conditions are presented in the categories of anemias and clotting disorders. The opening scenario of a child with sickle cell anemia is later applied to a fully developed nursing care plan for a child with this disorder. The chapter closes with a brief overview of bone marrow transplantation.

Learning Objectives

- Distinguish among the cells that make up the cellular portion of blood.
- Describe how sickle cell anemia is transmitted.
- Discuss the mechanism whereby the red blood cells become sickle-shaped in sickle cell anemia.
- Differentiate among the types of sickle cell crises.
- Outline the nursing management of a child in sickle cell crisis.
- Discuss the nursing management of the populations at risk for iron deficiency anemia.
- Describe the clinical manifestations of ß-thalassemia and aplastic anemia and the medical and nursing management of children with these disorders.
- Describe how hemophilia is transmitted.
- Discuss the clinical manifestations of hemophilia and other selected clotting disorders and the medical and nursing management of children with these disorders.
- Describe bone marrow transplantation and identify conditions for which it may be used.

Key Terms

anemia
ecchymosis
erythropoiesis
hemarthrosis
hematopoiesis
hemoglobinopathy
hemosiderosis
leukopenia
menorrhagia
pancytopenia
petechiae
polycythemia
purpura
thrombocytopenia
vaso-occlusion

Chapter Outline

Anatomy and Physiology of Pediatric Differences
    Red Blood Cells
    White Blood Cells
    Platelets
Anemias
    Iron Deficiency Anemia
        Nursing Management
    Normocytic Anemia
    Sickle Cell Anemia
        Clinical Manifestations
        Etiology and Pathophysiology
        Diagnostic Tests and Medical Management
        Nursing Assessment
        Nursing Diagnosis
        Nursing Management
ß-Thalassemia
    Nursing Management
Aplastic Anemia
    Nursing Management
Clotting Disorders
    Hemophilia
        Clinical Manifestations
        Etiology and Pathophysiology
        Diagnostic Tests and Medical Management
        Nursing Assessment
        Nursing Diagnosis
        Nursing Management
    Von Willebrand Disease
        Nursing Management
    Disseminated Intravascular Coagulation
        Nursing Management
    Idiopathic Thrombocytopenic Purpura
        Nursing Management
    Meningococcemia
        Nursing Management
Bone Marrow Transplantation

Tables

Overhead Transparency

Fig. 13-1   Type of blood cells (p. 517)

Audio-Visual Resources

1. *Blood.- The Microscopic Miracle*
Videocassette or 16 mm, 22 minutes
Source: Encyclopedia Britannica Educational Corporation
2. *Genetic Counseling*
Filmstrip, 19 minutes
Source: March of Dimes Birth Defects Foundation
3. *Matter of Chance* (Sickle Cell Anemia)
Videocassette, 28 minutes
Source: National Audio-Visual Center
4. *Blood Transfusion Today*
Videocassette, 58 minutes
Source: National Audio-Visual Center
5. *Living with Chronic Illness* (Hemophilia)
Videocassette, 29 minutes
Source: Public Television Library
6. *Joey* (Hemophilia)
16 mm, 18 minutes
Source: National Hemophilia Foundation
7. *Heredity and Hemophilia*
Slide-Audiocassette, 12 minutes
Source: Cutter Biological
8. *Inside a Bleeding Joint*
Slide-Audiocassette, 12 minutes
Source: Cutter Biological
9. *Home Infusion Techniques for Hemophiliacs*
Slide-Audiocassette, 20 minutes
Source: Abbott Scientific Products Division

Potential Problem Areas for Students

1. Students may not recall the patterns of heredity of the genetic disorders discussed in this chapter. Overhead transparencies that depict autosomal recessive and X-linked inheritance patterns would review and reinforce this information.

2. Students may have difficulty distinguishing among the various sickle cell disorders. An overhead transparency that lists the major attributes of each disorder could assist with this conceptualization.
3. It is often difficult for students to understand the pathophysiology of the various clotting disorders. A hand-out with a diagram of the clotting mechanisms that identifies the factors responsible for each disorder could clarify this material.

Activities to Foster Critical Thinking

A. CLASSROOM ACTIVITIES

1. Following the presentation of sickle cell anemia, divide students into two groups for discussion. Have one group take the position that sickle cell screening should be required as an essential component of pediatric health care and the other argue against this on grounds of personal choice and privacy.
2. Present a vignette of a child with a hematologic disorder who requires a blood transfusion. Have students identify:
   (a) potential problems for the child,
   (b) nursing responsibilities in the administration of blood products, and
   (c) parental concerns.
3. Invite a genetic counselor to speak to the class on the role of genetic counseling in the care of families with hereditary hematologic disorders. Focus post-presentation discussion on the role of the nurse in the referral and counseling process.
4. Invite a community nurse who cares for children with hematologic disorders to speak to the class about home management and community resources.

Have students discuss the ways in which nursing activities differ according to the care setting.
5. Have students interview parents of a child with a hematologic disorder regarding:
   (a) impact of the diagnosis,
   (b) impact of the management of the disorder on the child and family, and
   (c) parental evaluation of professional resources and support services.

B. CLINICAL ACTIVITIES

1. Assign students to care for a child with a congenital or acquired hematologic disorder and develop a nursing care plan for the child and family.
2. Have students examine the agency policies regarding blood administration. Ask them to identify ways in which these would protect a child receiving a blood transfusion.
3. Arrange for students to attend a hematology or hemophilia clinic and:
   (a) observe the role of the nurse in caring for children in these settings and
   (b) identify the developmental issues for these children.
4. Arrange for students to attend a support group meeting for families of children with hemophilia to determine issues raised and avenues of support.
5. Arrange for students to visit a genetic counseling center to observe protocols and identify issues that are commonly dealt with in the genetic counseling process.
6. Have students identify a learning need of a child and family with a hematologic disorder in a clinic, home, or acute care setting. Have them develop a teaching plan to meet this need.

14

ALTERATIONS IN CELLULAR GROWTH

Chapter Overview

Chapter 14 deals with the various childhood cancers, beginning with a general overview of cancer in children and their nursing care needs. It then discusses specific childhood cancers, including brain tumors, neuroblastoma, Wilms' tumor, bone tumors, leukemia, and soft tissue tumors. Nursing management of children with each of these cancers is emphasized. A nursing care plan for the home care of the child with cancer applies nursing management principles to the home setting.

Learning Objectives

• Explain the significance of the differences between adult and pediatric cancers.
• Describe the general etiology of cancer in children.
• Discuss the various therapies used to treat childhood cancer.
• Describe the effect of a child's cancer diagnosis on the family.
• Describe the nursing assessment and management of children undergoing treatment for cancer.
• Discuss the clinical manifestations of selected childhood cancers and their medical and nursing management.

Key Terms

benign
biotherapy
carcinogens
chemotherapy
extravasation
leukocytosis
leukopenia
malignant
metastasis
myelosuppression
neoplasms
oncogene
polypharmacy
protocol
protooncogene
radiation
thrombocytopenia
tumor suppressor genes

Chapter Outline

Anatomy and Physiology of Pediatric Differences
Childhood Cancer
    Incidence
    Clinical Manifestations
    Etiology and Pathophysiology
    Diagnostic Tests and Medical Management
    Nursing Assessment
    Nursing Diagnosis
    Nursing Management
Brain Tumors
    Clinical Manifestations and Pathophysiology

Tables

Overhead Transparencies

Audio-Visual Resources

1. *Nursing Management of Children with Cancer*
   Videocassette, 20 minutes
   Source: American Cancer Society
2. *Bone Marrows and Spinal Taps: A Child's View; Part 1: Danielle*
   Videocassette, 12 minutes
   Source: Carle Medical Communications
3. *Bone Marrows and Spinal Taps: A Child's View; Part IT Ronald*
   Videocassette, 12 minutes
   Source: Carle Medical Communications
4. *Bone Marrows, Spinal Taps and You*
   Videocassette, 19 minutes
   Source: M.D.A. TV

5. *People You'd Like to Know Series: Diana*
   16 mm, 10 minutes
   Source: Encyclopedia Britannica Educational Corporation

6. *Only One Road: Three Families Coping with Childhood Cancer*
   Videocassette, 53 minutes
   Source: University of Michigan

7. *ABC Close-up: Can't It Be Anyone Else?*
   Videocassette, 60 minutes
   Source: American Broadcasting Company

8. *Childhood Cancer*
   Videocassette, 59 minutes
   Source: Filmmaker's Library

9. *Coping with Cancer: The Early School Years*
   Videocassette, 36 minutes
   Source: American Journal of Nursing Co.

10. *Coping with Cancer: The Middle-School Years*
    Videocassette, 36 minutes
    Source: American Journal of Nursing Co.

11. *Coping with Cancer: The Sibling Perspective*
    Videocassette, 20 minutes
    Source: American Journal of Nursing Co.

12. *Caring for the Myelosuppressed Child*
    Videocassette with Study Guide, 28 minutes
    Source: American Journal of Nursing Co.

13. *Julie and John*
    Videocassette, *35* minutes
    Source: Health Sciences Consortium

14. *My Hair's Falling Out ... Am I Still Pretty?*
    Videocassette, 22 minutes
    Source: Association for the Care of Children's Health

15. *We Can Do It*
    Videocassette, 14 minutes
    Source: American Journal of Nursing Co.

Potential Problem Areas for Students

1. Students may find the experience of caring for a child with cancer emotionally overwhelming. Showing a recommended audio-visual program and discussing the issues raised prior to their clinical experience would allow students to examine their own feelings. This could prepare them to deal more adequately in the clinical area with the child and family affected by cancer.

2. Students tend to think of leukemia in terms of white blood cell proliferation without understanding the accompanying bone marrow depression and depletion of cellular elements. A brief review of hematopoiesis that is linked to the explanation of the pathophysiology of leukemia could be helpful in promoting the understanding of leukemia's underlying mechanisms and clinical manifestations.

Activities to Foster Critical Thinking

A. CLASSROOM ACTIVITIES

1. Show a recommended audio-visual program and focus discussion on:
   (a) the developmental and psychological issues it raises for the child and
   (b) the nursing support needed by the entire family.

2. Invite a staff nurse or home care nurse experienced in caring for children with cancer to speak to the class regarding this nursing role. Ask students to share their feelings and concerns about such a position.

3. Present a vignette of a preschool-age child with acute lymphocytic leukemia. Ask students to write down:
   (a) their major concern if they were assigned to care for this child,
   (b) one psychosocial nursing intervention for the child, and
   (c) one support measure for the family. Use responses for class discussion.

B. CLINICAL ACTIVITIES

1. Arrange for students to spend a day in the pediatric oncology clinic or follow the pediatric oncology nurse specialist to observe protocols. Discuss observations related to the nurse's role and children's responses.

2. Assign students to care for a child with cancer in an acute care or home setting. Require that a nursing care plan be developed for the child and family.

3. Have students develop a teaching plan for a child who will be:
   (a) having a spinal tap or bone marrow aspiration or
   (b) receiving radiation or chemotherapy. Utilize agency protocols and the child's age as the basis for developing this plan.

4. Assign students to interview a child with cancer or a family member regarding:
   (a) the impact of the diagnosis,
   (b) coping strategies, and
   (c) reactions to care.
   Discuss responses in clinical conference.

5. Arrange for students to attend a support group for children with cancer or leukemia or for their families. Ask them to identify concerns raised and types of support provided.

ALTERATIONS IN GASTROINTESTINAL FUNCTION

Chapter Overview

Chapter 15 offers a detailed description of gastrointestinal disorders in children, after first identifying this system's variations during infancy and childhood. Conditions are grouped for discussion as structural defects, hernias, inflammatory disorders, disorders of motility, parasitic disorders, feeding disorders, and injuries. The pre- and postoperative care of ostomies is described. Two nursing care plans—one for care of the child with a cleft lip and/or palate, and one for care of the child with gastroenteritis—apply the material to clinical practice.

Learning Objectives

- Identify significant differences between the adult and pediatric GI systems.
- Compare and contrast the structural defects that cause dysfunction in the GI system.
- Describe the nursing management of children with cleft lip and/or palate defects.
- Formulate discharge instructions for children following cleft lip repair.
- Describe the clinical manifestations of various structural disorders that cause GI obstruction and the medical and nursing management of children with these disorders.
- Describe the care of children with diaphragmatic or umbilical hernias.
- Discuss the nursing assessment and management of children with inflammatory disorders of the GI system.
- Discuss the impact of an ostomy on the growth and development of an adolescent.
- Describe the nursing management of children with motility disorders.
- Describe the transmission and clinical manifestations of common intestinal parasites.
- Describe the anticipatory guidance needed for children with feeding and malabsorptive disorders.
- Discuss the nursing assessment and management of children with hepatic disorders.
- Recognize the effects of common toxic agents and describe the treatment of children poisoned by these agents.
- Discuss common abdominal injuries that can occur in children.

Key Terms

cholestasis
constipation
deamination
diarrhea
gluconeogenesis
hernia
occult blood
ostomy
peristalsis
projectile vomiting

Chapter Outline

Tables

15-1 Parent Teaching: Home Care Instructions for the Child Requiring Gastrostomy Tube Feedings and Care

15-2 Medications Used to Treat Gastroesophageal Reflux

15-3 Management of Anorectal Malformations

15-4 Comparison of Ulcerative Colitis and Crohn's Disease

15-5 Drugs used in Treatment of Inflammatory Bowel Disease

15-6 Causes of Diarrhea in Children

15-7 Treatment of Diarrhea

15-8 Common Intestinal Parasitic Disorders

15-9 Parent Teaching: Suggestions for Alleviating Colic

15-10 Comparison of Hepatitis Types

15-11 Transmission, Immunization, and Prophylaxis for Hepatitis

15-12 Treatment for Complications of Cirrhosis

15-13 Commonly Ingested Toxic Agents

15-14 Emergency Management for Poisoning

15-15 Sources of Lead Exposure

15-16 Clinical Manifestations of Lead Poisoning

Audio-Visual Resources

1. *How to Feed Your Baby Who Has a Cleft Lip or Palate*
   Slide/tape, 11 minutes
   Source: Health Sciences Consortium

2. *Insertion of an Infant Gavage Feeding Tube*
   Videocassette, 11 minutes
   Source: Ross Laboratories

3. *Ostomy Care*
   Videocassette, 13 minutes
   Source: Health Sciences Consortium

4. *Your Child's Ostomy*
   Videocassette, 12 minutes
   Source: American Journal of Nursing Co.

5. *Living with Inflammatory Bowel Disease*
   16 mm, 15 minutes
   Source: National Foundation for Ileitis and Colitis, Inc.

6. *Long-Term Central Venous Catheters for Pediatric Patients*
   Videocassette with Study Guide, 28 minutes
   Source: American Journal of Nursing Co.

7. *Close to the Heart, Part T A Discussion About Central Venous Lines*
   Videocassette, 15 minutes
   Source: American Journal of Nursing Co.

8. *Close to the Heart, Part 1I—Heparinization and Emergency Care of Central Lines*
   Videocassette, 30 minutes
   Source: American Journal of Nursing Co.

Potential Problem Areas for Students

1. Students need to be aware of the potential for metabolic acid–base imbalances and fluid and electrolyte imbalances in children with most gastrointestinal disorders. A review of this material prior to beginning the unit could help with appropriate application.

2. Students may have difficulty grasping the differences between Crohn's disease and ulcerative colitis. An overhead transparency that compare the conditions in terms of area of bowel affected, tissue differences, clinical manifestations, and management could help with differentiation.

3. Students may not be knowledgeable about special pediatric considerations when central venous catheters are utilized for fluid and nutritional maintenance. Viewing one of the recommended audio-visual programs could enhance students' ability to care for a child with a central line and provide support for the parents.

Activities to Foster Critical Thinking

A. CLASSROOM ACTIVITIES

1. Show one of the recommended audio-visual programs that focuses on a nursing procedure related to the gastrointestinal system. Have the class identify:
   (a) ways in which the procedure is similar for the adult and child,
   (b) pediatric differences in the procedure, and
   (c) nursing strategies to increase the child's comfort during the procedure.

2. Invite a nurse practitioner who works with children with gastrointestinal disorders to speak to the class about this nursing role. Have each student submit a question for the speaker in advance.

3. Invite a pediatric dietitian to speak to the class about nutritional management in gastrointestinal conditions during childhood. Have students identify ways in which nurses can support this management.

4. Present local statistics on lead poisoning to the class. Ask students to:
   (a) identify potential sources of lead for children,
   (b) list characteristics that place children at risk, and
   (c) describe nursing responsibilities related to prevention, treatment, and follow-up.

5. Invite a representative from the local Poison Control Center to speak to the class on the center's activities. Focus discussion on nursing responsibilities in prevention of and emergency response to poisonings.

B. CLINICAL ACTIVITIES

1. Assign students to care for a child with any of the gastrointestinal disorders presented in this chapter and develop a comprehensive nursing care plan for the child and family.

2. Arrange for students to visit one of the following: pediatric clinic, pediatric gastroenterology clinic, lead clinic, or pediatric surgeon's office. At clinical conference, discuss the disorders observed, reactions of the child and parents to services, and the observed nursing role in each setting.

3. Arrange for students to attend a support group meeting for children with gastrointestinal disorders and their families. Have students discuss the issues raised and support services accessed.

4. Assign students to assess a teaching need in a child and family with a gastrointestinal disorder. Require students to develop, implement, and evaluate a teaching plan to meet this need.

5. Assign students to interview a parent of a child with a chronic gastrointestinal disorder to determine the impact of the diagnosis and ongoing care on the family.

16

ALTERATIONS IN GENITOURINARY FUNCTION

Chapter Overview

Chapter 16 addresses disorders of the reproductive, renal, and urinary systems during childhood, citing first the pediatric differences in these systems. Disorders are discussed in the categories of structural defects, urinary tract infections, enuresis, renal disorders, and sexually transmitted diseases. A nursing care plan for a child with acute poststreptococcal glomerulonephritis provides an application of the concepts of nursing management.

Learning Objectives

- Identify the differences between the adult and pediatric genitourinary systems.
- Describe selected structural defects of the urinary and reproductive systems and the medical and nursing management of children with these defects.
- Identify the cause of most urinary tract infections.
- Discuss the treatment of urinary tract infections and describe an educational plan to prevent future infections in children of various ages.

- Describe enuresis and the medical and nursing management of children with this disorder.
- Explain the etiology of selected renal disorders and the medical and nursing management of children with these disorders.
- Differentiate between hemodialysis and peritoneal dialysis.
- Differentiate among selected sexually transmitted diseases.
- Describe the educational plan for an adolescent diagnosed with a sexually transmitted disease.

Key Terms

azotemia
dialysate
end-stage renal disease
enuresis
hydronephrosis
oliguria
osteodystrophy
Renal insufficiency
stent
uremia
vesicoureteral reflux

Chapter Outline

Tables

Audio-Visual Resources

1. *Obtaining and Culturing Urine*
   Videocassette, 14 minutes
   Source: Health Sciences Consortium
2. *Obtaining a Clean Catch Urine Specimen*
   Videocassette, 9 minutes
   Source: Health Sciences Consortium
3. *New Concepts in Urinary Tract Infections*
   16 mm, 15 minutes
   Source: Vacumate Corporation
4. *Anatomy of the Kidneys, Ureters, and Bladder*
   Slide/tape, 15 minutes
   Source: Trainex Corporation
5. *Physiology of the Kidneys*
   Slide/tape, 15 minutes
   Source: Trainex Corporation
6. *Dialysis: An Overview*
   Slidetape: 14 minutes
   Source: Trainex Corporation
7. *Life without Kidneys: A Second Chance at Living*
   16 mm, 15 minutes
   Source: NAPHT, Inc.
8. *Venereal Disease: The Hidden Epidemic*
   16 mm, 27 minutes
   Source: Encyclopedia Britannica Educational Corporation
9. *Half a Million Teenagers*
   16 mm, 20 minutes
   Source: Churchill Films

Potential Problem Areas for Students

1. Students may have difficulty differentiating between nephrotic syndrome and glomerulonephritis because they do not relate underlying pathophysiology to the clinical manifestations. A chart that compares the two disorders in terms of pathophysiology, etiology, age group, clinical manifestations, and management could resolve this difficulty.
2. Students may not recognize the potential conflicts between children's and parents' rights in situations involving sexually transmitted diseases in the pediatric and adolescent population. A review of policies related to informed consent and confidentiality specific to the laws of the state could make students aware of both potential conflicts and policies for their resolution.

Activities to Foster Critical Thinking

A. CLASSROOM ACTIVITIES

1. Present vignettes of two preschool-age children, one with acute poststreptococcal glomerulonephritis and one with nephrotic syndrome. Ask students to compare:
   (a) pathophysiology,
   (b) clinical manifestations, and
   (c) medical and nursing management.
2. Invite a dialysis nurse to speak to the class about this nursing role. Focus class discussion around:
   (a) special problems related to dialysis of the pediatric patient,
   (b) the child's and family's reactions to dialysis, and
   (c) home versus hospital-based dialysis programs.
3. Invite a home care nurse experienced in the care of children with genitourinary disorders to speak to the class about the home nursing management of these children. Have students discuss the advantages and disadvantages of the home setting for this care.
4. Present a vignette of a child in chronic renal failure who is awaiting a donor kidney for transplantation surgery. Ask students to discuss the impact of waiting and the actual surgery on the child and family.
5. Present the local statistics on the various sexually transmitted diseases. Ask students to discuss the factors that contribute to the increase in adolescents with STI)s and the potential sequelae of these disorders.

B. CLINICAL ACTIVITIES

1. Assign students to care for a child or adolescent with a genitourinary disorder and develop a comprehensive nursing care plan based on an assessment of the child's status.
2. Assign students to develop, implement, and evaluate a teaching plan for a child or adolescent with one of the following:

(a) urinary tract infection,

(b) dialysis,

(c) anticipated kidney transplant, or

(d) a sexually transmitted disease.

3. Arrange for students to attend a children's renal clinic to observe the types of conditions managed, the treatments utilized, reactions of the child, and role of the nurse.

4. Arrange for students to observe in a dialysis unit. Have them:

(a) compare and contrast adult and pediatric protocols,

(b) identify problems encountered with children in this setting, and

(c) analyze the role of the nurse.

5. Assign students to interview a child receiving dialysis to determine the child's feelings about the procedure and its impact on lifestyle. At clinical conference, ask students to suggest nursing interventions to minimize the impact of this procedure on children.

17

ALTERATIONS IN EYE, EAR, NOSE, AND THROAT FUNCTION

Chapter Overview

Chapter 17 describes common childhood conditions that affect functioning of the eyes, ears, nose, and throat. It opens with a discussion of important childhood differences in these structures. Following presentation of various disorders and their management, this chapter focuses on visual and hearing impairments in children. Nursing care plans for the child with otitis media and the child undergoing tonsillectomy provide application to commonly encountered childhood situations.

Learning Objectives

- Identify normal variations in the eye, ear, nose, and throat in the pediatric population.
- Discuss medical and nursing management of children with infections of the eye.
- Describe selected visual disorders and their treatment.
- Describe the clinical manifestations of children with visual impairments.
- Discuss the emergency care of children with selected eye injuries.
- Summarize the etiology of otitis media and the medical and nursing management of children with this disorder.
- Describe the clinical manifestations of children with hearing impairments.

- Differentiate between conductive and sensorineural hearing loss.
- Discuss the emergency care of children with selected ear injuries.
- Describe the nursing assessment and management of children with epistaxis.
- Describe the medical and nursing management of children with strep throat and tonsillitis.

Key Terms

audiography
binocularity
conductive hearing loss
decibels
mixed hearing loss
myringotomy
sensorineural hearing loss
tympanogram
tympanotomy tubes
visual acuity
vision

Chapter Outline

Anatomy and Physiology of Pediatric Differences
    Eye
    Ear
    Nose and Throat

Tables

Audio-Visual Resources

1. *Amblyopia*
Videocassette, 7 minutes
Source: American Journal of Nursing Co.
2. *Esotropia*
Videocassette, 7 minutes
Source: American Journal of Nursing Co.
3. *Exotropia*
Videocassette, 6 minutes
Source: American Journal of Nursing Co.
4. *Eye Trauma*
Videocassette, 28 minutes
Source: American Journal of Nursing Co.
5. *Before We Are Six*
16 mm, 20 minutes
Source: National Society to Prevent Blindness

6. *Acute Middle Ear Disease in Infants and Children*
   Slide-Audiocassette, 22 minutes
   Source: National Audio-Visual Center
7. *Can Your Patient Hear?*
   Videocassette, 32 minutes
   Source: Health Sciences Consortium
8. *The Day of Jasper's Operation* (Tonsillectomy)
   Videocassette, 14 minutes
   Source: Kid's Comer
9. *People You'd Like to Know: Harold* (Visual Impairment)
   16 mm, 10 minutes
   Source: Encyclopedia Brittannica. Educational Corporation
10. *Sound of Sunshine, Sound of Rain* (Visual Impairment)
    Videocassette, 14 minutes
    Source: Film Fair Communications
11. *Language and Hearing Impaired Children*
    Videocassette, 15 minutes
    Source: Health Sciences Consortium
12. *My Perfect Child Is Deaf*
    Videocassette or 16 mm, 30 minutes
    Source: Pyramid Film and Video
13. *What Do I Do Now?* (Hearing Impairment)
    Videocassette or 16 mm, 30 minutes
    Source: Pyramid Film and Video
14. *What Can My Child Hear?*
    Videocassette or 16 mm, 30 minutes
    Source: Pyramid Film and Video
15. *Like Me Series: Everyone Needs Some Help* (Hearing Impairment)
    16 mm, 7 minutes
    Source: Encyclopedia Britannica, Educational Corporation

Potential Problem Areas for Students

1. Students may not be aware of how the anatomical and physiological variations in the eyes, ears, nose, and throat of a child influence the development of common childhood disorders. An overhead transparency that lists these differences with their potential impact would make this information clear.
2. Students may encounter children with sensory impairments in a variety of settings and hesitate to communicate with them. Showing a recommended

audio-visual program that deals with this problem and discussing the techniques observed prior to the student clinical experience could facilitate the communication process.

Activities to Foster Critical Thinking

A. CLASSROOM ACTIVITIES

1. Invite a school nurse to speak to the class about the nurse's role in screening for visual and hearing problems in the school setting. Following the presentation, ask students to describe problems that might be encountered and benefits to the child.
2. Show a recommended audio-visual program about visual or hearing impairment and ask students to identify:
   (a) their feelings about sensory impairments,
   (b) societal issues related,
   (c) communication barriers, and
   (d) strategies that could be used with children for overcoming these barriers.

B. CLINICAL ACTIVITIES

1. Assign students to care for a child with a condition of the eye, ear, nose, or throat and develop a nursing care plan for the child and family.
2. Arrange for students to follow a child coming to the hospital for a tonsillectomy from admission to discharge. Require the students to develop, implement, and evaluate both pre- and postoperative teaching plans with the child and family.
3. Arrange for students to participate in the vision and hearing screenings in an educational setting. Have students identify:
   (a) the nurse's role in the process in the specific setting,
   (b) problems encountered in the screening process,
   (c) what kind of vision and hearing problems were found, and
   (d) procedures for following up on identified problems.
4. Arrange for students to observe activities in a children's speech and hearing center. Ask students to describe:

(a) activities observed,

(b) problems identified at each developmental stage, and

(c) roles that nursing could play in managing problems found.

5. Arrange for students to visit a school for visually or hearing impaired children and observe approaches to communication and instruction. Ask them to compare and contrast this environment with a public school setting.

ALTERATIONS IN NEUROLOGIC FUNCTION

Chapter Overview

Chapter 18 presents a comprehensive view of neurologic disorders in children. It provides a conceptual base by identifying pediatric neurologic differences and discussing methods for assessing levels of consciousness and general neurologic status. Neurologic disorders are addressed in the categories of seizure disorders, infectious diseases, drug-addicted infants, cerebral palsy, and neurologic injuries. A nursing care plan for a child with bacterial meningitis provides application of the material to a clinical situation.

Learning Objectives

- Identify significant differences between the adult and pediatric nervous systems.
- Describe the assessment of level of consciousness.
- Describe the use of selected neurologic assessment tools.
- Identify signs of increased intracranial pressure.
- Discuss care of the immobile child.
- Discuss the clinical manifestations of selected seizure disorders and the medical and nursing management of children with these disorders.
- Describe selected infectious diseases that have neurologic implications in children.
- Describe the anatomy and clinical manifestations of selected structural defects of the neurologic system and the medical and nursing management of children with these defects.
- Discuss identification and care of the infant experiencing neonatal abstinence syndrome.
- Describe the clinical manifestations of cerebral palsy and the medical and nursing management of children with this disorder.
- Describe the etiology, clinical manifestations, and medical and nursing management of head injuries in children.
- Discuss the medical and nursing management of children who have experienced spinal cord injury or near drowning.

Key Terms

areflexia
aura
cerebral edema
cerebral perfusion pressure
clonic
coma
confusion
Cushing's triad
delirium
encephalopathy
focal

intracranial pressure
level of consciousness
obtunded
postictal period
posturing
stupor
tonic

Chapter Outline

Tables

Overhead Transparencies

Audio-Visual Resources

1. *Neurological Assessment of the Pediatric Patient*
   Videocassette with Study Guide, 28 minutes
   Source: American Journal of Nursing Co.
2. *Assessing Levels of Consciousness: The Glasgow Coma Scale*
   Videocassette, 7 minutes
   Source: Health Sciences Consortium
3. *Nursing Management of Increased Intracranial Pressure*
   Videocassette, 10 minutes
   Source: American Journal of Nursing Co.
4. *Seizure and Movement Disorders in Children*
   Videocassette, 26 minutes
   Source: Ross Laboratories
5. *Like You, Like Me Series: Let's Talk It Over* (Seizures)
   16 mm, 6 minutes
   Source: Encyclopedia Britannica Educational Corporation
6. *Understanding Spina Bifida*
   Videocassette, 20 minutes
   Source: University of Kansas Medical Center
7. *Just Like Me? Children Talk About Spina Bifida*
   Videocassette, 14 minutes
   Source: New England Regional Genetics Group (NERGG)
8. *Teaching Children with Spina Bifida*
   Videocassette, *30* minutes
   Source: Paul H. Brookes Publishing Company
9. *Cerebral Palsy*
   Videocassette, 12 minutes
   Source: Health Sciences Consortium
10. *Nursing Management of Acute Head Injuries*
    Videocassette, 28 minutes
    Source: American Journal of Nursing Co.
11. *Complications of Spinal Cord Impairment*
    Videocassette, 28 minutes
    Source: American Journal of Nursing Co.
12. *Robbie: A Teenage Quadriplegic*
    Videocassette or 16 mm, *30* minutes
    Source: American Journal of Nursing Co.

Potential Problem Areas for Students

1. Students tend to memorize material related to assessment of neurologic status without understanding the reasons for neurologic changes. Overhead transparencies that review the regulatory mechanisms of the brain and age-related variations would serve as a starting point for relating neurologic changes to significant observations.
2. Student conceptualization of seizure disorders may be restricted to generalized grand mal episodes. A hand-out that lists the various forms of seizures by type and manifestations could make this material clearer and more meaningful.
3. Students often do not understand why spina bifida presents with such a wide variation in symptoms from child to child. Use of a diagram that relates the level of the lesion to the distribution of the spinal nerves affected could clarify this area.

Activities to Foster Critical Thinking

A. CLASSROOM ACTIVITIES

1. Show one of the recommended audio-visual programs on a neurologic disorder in children. Focus discussion on identification of issues and nursing roles and actions.
2. Invite a physical therapist who works with children to speak to the class about therapies used with children with spina bifida, cerebral palsy, head injuries, or spinal cord injuries. Ask students how nurses working with these children can complement these therapies.
3. Invite a school nurse to speak to the class about caring for children with neurologic disorders within the school setting. Have students identify:
   (a) the various components of the school nursing role,
   (b) the problems that children with neurologic disorders may encounter in the school setting, and
   (c) strategies to assist them in overcoming these problems.

B. CLINICAL ACTIVITIES

1. Assign students to care for a child with a neurologic disorder. Require that a comprehensive nursing care plan be developed, based on the findings of a careful assessment of the child's status.
2. Arrange for students to visit a neurology, seizure, spina bifida, cerebral palsy, head injury, or spinal cord injury clinic for children. Have them report on:
   (a) specific clinical activities,
   (b) the role of the nurse in the clinical setting, and
   (c) observed reactions of the child and family to services delivered.
3. Arrange for students to attend a support group for parents of children with a specific neurologic disorder to identify the issues raised and avenues of support. Have students compare and contrast the groups and their concerns in clinical conference.
4. Arrange for students to observe activities related to management of a child's neurologic disorder in one of the following settings: emergency room, PICU, operating room, physical therapy department, home, or school. In each setting, have them identify the nurse's role.
5. Have students develop, implement, and evaluate a family teaching plan for a childhood neurologic disorder.

19

ALTERATIONS IN
MUSCULOSKELETAL FUNCTION

Chapter Overview

Chapter 19 discusses the various conditions that represent an alteration in musculoskeletal function during childhood. The pediatric differences in bones, muscles, tendons, and ligaments are briefly described. The specific musculoskeletal disorders are presented within the classifications of disorders of the feet and legs, disorders of the hip, disorders of the spine, disorders of the bones and joints, muscular dystrophies, and injuries to the system. A nursing care plan for a child undergoing surgery for scoliosis provides a synthesis of nursing management principles for clinical practice.

Learning Objectives

- Identify the differences between the adult and pediatric musculoskeletal systems.
- Discuss the clinical manifestations of children with selected disorders of the feet and legs and the medical and nursing care of children with these disorders.
- Describe the clinical manifestations of developmental dysplasia of the hip and the medical and nursing management of children with this disorder.
- Discuss the clinical manifestations of selected acquired disorders of the hip and the medical and nursing management of children with these disorders.

- Identify the classic signs of scoliosis.
- Describe the medical and nursing management of adolescents with scoliosis.
- Discuss the medical and nursing management of children with infections of the bones and joints.
- Describe the genetic transmission and clinical manifestations of osteogenesis imperfecta, and the medical and nursing management of children with this disorder.
- Discuss the genetic transmission and clinical manifestations of selected muscular dystrophies and the medical and nursing management of children with these disorders.
- Discuss the clinical manifestations and nursing management of selected injuries to the musculoskeletal system.
- Describe the care of children in casts and traction.

Key Terms

chondrolysis
dislocation
dysplasia
equinus
ossification
osteotomy
pseudohypertrophy
subluxation
varus

Chapter Outline

Tables

Overhead Transparencies

Tab. 19-1   Musculoskeletal positions (p. 818)
Tab. 19-13   Classification and types of fractures (p. 854)
Fig. 19-18   The Salter-Harris classification of fractures (p. 855)

Audio-Visual Resources

1. *Orthopedic Assessment*
   Videocassette, 28 minutes
   Source: American Journal of Nursing Co.
2. *Child with Orthopedic Anomalies*
   16 mm, 16 minutes
   Source: Prentice-Hall, Inc.
3. *Nursing Care of Patients with Casts*
   Videocassette, 28 minutes
   Source: American Journal of Nursing Co.
4. *Caring for the Child in a Hip Spica Cast*
   Slide/Audiocassette, 19 minutes
   Source: University of Michigan
5. *Early Detection of Scoliosis*
   Videocassette, 9 minutes
   Source: Health Sciences Consortium
6. *Scoliosis*
   Videocassette, 30 minutes
   Source: Health Sciences Consortium
7. *Spinal Fusion: What You Need to Know*
   Videocassette, 18 minutes
   Source: University of Michigan
8. *Muscular Dystrophy and Related Diseases: A Differential Diagnosis*
   Videocassette, 32 minutes
   Source: National Audio-Visual Center
9. *A Broken Nose*
   16 mm, 25 minutes
   Source: Fairview General Hospital
10. *Principles of Traction*
    16 mm, 20 minutes
    Source: Fairview General Hospital
11. *Children in Traction*
    Videocassette, 27 minutes
    Source: Fairview General Hospital
12. *Krista*
    16 mm, 20 minutes
    Source: Child, Youth and Family Services

Potential Problem Areas for Students

1. Much of the terminology related to the musculoskeletal disorders is specific to the orthopedic specialty and may be unfamiliar to students. Providing a glossary of terms could help familiarize students with this area and allow them to focus on the underlying principles of pathophysiology and management.
2. Students may not understand the mechanisms of muscular dystrophy that are the root of the clinical manifestations observed. A review of neuromuscular physiology that is linked to the functional changes seen in the muscular dystrophies could promote a clearer understanding.
3. Many students have difficulty understanding the principles of physics as they apply to traction and realignment of fractures. Providing an overhead transparency that diagrams the directional forces of the basic types of traction could promote better understanding of this area.

Activities to Foster Critical Thinking

A. CLASSROOM ACTIVITIES

1. Assign groups of students to develop presentations on the following:
   (a) care of a preschool child in a cast,
   (b) care of a school-age child in traction, and
   (c) care of an adolescent following surgery to correct scoliosis.
2. Invite a staff nurse who is experienced in the care of children with musculoskeletal disorders to speak to the class about this nursing role. Focus discussion on nursing interventions to support normal development in children with casts, in traction, or with a chronic limitation of mobility.
3. Invite a physical therapist to speak to the class about use of orthoses, crutch walking, and various therapies for children with musculoskeletal disorders. Have the class discuss ways in which nursing activities can support and enhance the goals of these therapies.

B. CLINICAL ACTIVITIES

1. Assign students to care for a child with a disorder of the musculoskeletal system. Require that they develop a comprehensive nursing care plan based on the child's assessed needs.

2. Assign students to develop, implement and evaluate a teaching plan for a child in a cast or in traction and the family.

3. Arrange for students to follow a child life specialist and observe the techniques used with children who are immobilized with a musculoskeletal disorder. Have students note:

(a) therapeutic play activities used,

(b) any adaptations made for immobility or assistive devices, and

(c) developmental consideration applied.

4. Arrange for students to observe the treatment of children in the physical therapy area. Have students note:

(a) types of therapy,

(b) teaching techniques, and

(c) responses of the children.

5. Arrange for students to visit the cast room and brace shop to observe cast application and removal as well as the various orthopedic devices used with children.

ALTERATIONS IN ENDOCRINE FUNCTION

Chapter Overview

Chapter 20 describes the complex conditions that result from altered endocrine function in children. The anatomy and physiology of pediatric endocrine differences are presented from the period of embryonic development through puberty. Disorders are grouped for discussion according to those resulting from altered functioning of the pituitary, thyroid, parathyroid, adrenals, pancreas, and gonads. In addition, disorders related to sex chromosome abnormalities and inborn errors of metabolism are presented. A nursing care plan for the child with newly diagnosed diabetes mellitus applies the material to the most common of the endocrine disorders in children.

Learning Objectives

- Discuss the role of various organs and glands of the endocrine system in the growth and development of children.
- Describe the etiology and clinical manifestations of selected disorders of the endocrine system.
- Discuss the medical and nursing management of children with selected endocrine disorders.
- Outline the medical and nursing management of children with insulin-dependent diabetes mellitus (IDDM).
- Describe the clinical manifestations of sex chromosome abnormalities and the medical and nursing management of children with these disorders.
- Identify disorders for which newborn screening is mandated.
- Describe the clinical manifestations of inborn errors of metabolism and the medical and nursing management of children with these disorders.

Key Terms

glucagon
glycosuria
goiter
hormone
Inborn errors of metabolism
karyotype
polydipsia
polyphagia
polyuria
pseudohermaphroditism
puberty

Chapter Outline

Anatomy and Physiology of Pediatric Differences
Disorders of Pituitary Function
    Hypopituitarism (Growth Hormone Deficiency)
        Nursing Management
    Hyperpituitarism
        Nursing Management

Tables

Overhead Transparencies

Audio-Visual Resources

1. *Evaluation of the Child with Small Stature*
   Videocassette, 27 minutes
   Source: University of Michigan
2. *Juvenile Diabetes: One Family's Story*
   Videocassette, 23 minutes
   Source: Health Sciences Consortium
3. *Survival Skills for Diabetic Children*
   Videocassette with Study Guide, 28 minutes
   Source: American Journal of Nursing Co.

4. *Amy—An Adolescent with Diabetes*
   Slide/tape, 15 minutes
   Source: University of Michigan
5. *Diabetic Ketoacidosis: Management in Children*
   Slide/tape, 27 minutes
   Source: University of Michigan
6. *Listen to the Kid—Adolescents Talk About Diabetes*
   Videocassette, 15 minutes
   Source: University of Michigan
7. *Self-Monitoring: Glucose and Ketones*
   Videocassette, 22 minutes
   Source: MedCom/Trainex
8. *Insulin Use and Management*
   Slide/tape, 22 minutes
   Source: MedCom/Trainex
9. *Hypoglycemia*
   Slide/tape, 38 minutes
   Source: University of Arizona
10. *Screening and Treatment of PKU*
    Slide/tape, 45 minutes
    Source: Health Sciences Consortium
11. *Carbohydrate Intolerance in Infancy*
    16 mm, 16 minutes
    Source: Ross Laboratories

Potential Problem Areas for Students

1. Students may not recognize the specific effects of hormonal abnormalities because of insufficient knowledge about hormonal functions. A series of overhead transparencies that present the major endocrine glands, hormones, and hormonal functions could provide the needed knowledge base.
2. Students may not be able to connect the clinical manifestations of diabetes mellitus to the underlying pathophysiology. Overhead transparencies that depict the role of insulin in glucose metabolism and the body's responses to insulin deficiency could help.

Activities to Foster Critical Thinking

A. CLASSROOM ACTIVITIES

1. Show one of the audio-visual programs on diabetes. Have students discuss the impact of the condition on the child's lifestyle and nursing interventions to minimize this impact.
2. Invite a pediatric dietitian to speak to the class about nutritional management of diabetes mellitus, hypoglycemia, and the inborn errors of metabolism in children. Focus class discussion on developmental issues and nursing actions to support nutritional management.
3. Invite a nurse who specializes in diabetic teaching to speak to the class about teaching children newly diagnosed with diabetes. Assign students to develop a teaching plan for a child and family, based on this presentation.
4. Invite a genetic counselor to speak to the class about the role of genetic counseling in families with an endocrine or metabolic disorder. Have students discuss the issues raised for these families and the nurse's role in supporting them.

B. CLINICAL ACTIVITIES

1. Assign students to care for a child with an endocrine or metabolic disorder and develop a comprehensive care plan for the child and family, based on an assessment of status.
2. Assign students to develop, implement, and evaluate a teaching plan for a child and family with an endocrine or metabolic disorder related to one of the following:
   (a) home monitoring,
   (b) dietary management, or
   (c) home medication administration.
3. Arrange for students to visit a pediatric endocrine or diabetic clinic to observe the management of these disorders. Ask students to identify:
   (a) reactions of the child and family and
   (b) the role of the nurse.
4. Assign students to interview the parents of a child who has had an endocrine or metabolic disorder for more than a year. Have them determine:
   (a) the initial impact of the condition and
   (b) concerns that have emerged in the course of home management of the child.
5. Arrange for students to follow a pediatric dietitian or child life specialist working with children with an endocrine or metabolic disorder. Have students discuss their observations at clinical conference related to activities observed and children's responses.

ALTERATIONS IN SKIN INTEGRITY

Chapter Overview

Chapter 21 introduces the groups of disorders related to alterations in skin integrity. After initially addressing the pediatric differences in the skin and its glands, the chapter discusses the basic types of skin lesions and the process of wound healing. It then presents a variety of skin disorders in the categories of dermatitis, infectious disorders, cellulitis, folliculitis, acne, and injuries to the skin. Two nursing care plans apply nursing management principles to the adolescent with acne and the child with a burn injury.

Learning Objectives

- Identify the differences between the skin of children and adults.
- Describe common secondary skin lesions.
- Discuss the care of children with dermatitis.
- Describe the cutaneous responses that occur in adverse reactions to drugs.
- Outline an educational plan for a child with eczema.
- Describe the medical and nursing management of children with selected infectious skin disorders.
- Discuss the care of children with cellulitis.
- Differentiate between folliculitis and acne and summarize the care of children with these disorders.
- Describe the medical and nursing management of selected injuries to the skin.
- List the types of burns and the classification of burn severity.
- Calculate the percentage of burn injury using a body surface area chart.
- Discuss the medical and nursing management of a child with major burns.

Key Terms

atopy
debridement
dermatophytoses
eschar
escharotomy
lichenification

Chapter Outline

Anatomy and Physiology of Pediatric Differences
Skin Lesions
Wound Healing
Dermatitis
    Contact Dermatitis
        Nursing Management
    Diaper Dermatitis
        Nursing Management
    Seborrheic Dermatitis
        Nursing Management

Tables

Overhead Transparencies

Audio-Visual Resources

1. *The Integumentary System*
   Videocassette, 22 minutes
   Source: MedCom/Trainex
2. *The Skin: Its Structure and Function*
   Videocassette or 16 mm, 20 minutes
   Source: Encyclopedia Britannica Educational Corporation
3. *Skin Rashes in Infants and Children*
   Programmed Instruction Package
   Source: American Journal of Nursing Co.
4. *Lice Are Not Nice*
   16 mm, 11 minutes
   Source: AIMS Media
5. *The Burned Child*
   16 mm, 44 minutes
   Source: Prentice-Hall, Inc.
6. *Here's Looking at You, Kid*
   16 mm, 53 minutes
   Source: Biomed Arts Associates, Inc.
7. *Nursing Care of Burn Patients: Part I, The First 72 Hours*
   Videocassette, 45 minutes
   Source: American Journal of Nursing Co.
8. *Nursing Care of Burn Patients: Part II, The Intermediate Phase*
   Videocassette, 45 minutes
   Source: American Journal of Nursing Co.
9. *The Other Child: Burns in Children*
   Videocassette, 50 minutes
   Source: American Journal of Nursing Co.

Potential Problem Areas for Students

1. Students tend to focus on the highly visible local reaction and may not understand the systemic responses to burn injuries. An overhead transparency that links the local response to hematologic changes and fluid and electrolyte shifts could promote understanding of the systemic responses involved and the reasons for their occurrence.
2. Students may think of burn severity only in terms of the depth of the burn. An overhead transparency could be useful in presenting assessment of pediatric burn severity. This should include a chart for determining the percentage of body surface area in

a child's burn injury, the relative percentages of some areas affected by growth, and specific burn distributions that increase severity.

Activities to Foster Critical Thinking

A. Classroom Activities

1. Invite a nurse from a dermatology clinic to speak to the class about skin disorders in children. Focus class discussion on nursing management techniques for the various developmental stages and the nurse's role in the clinic situation.
2. Invite a pediatric nurse practitioner to speak to the class about assessment of skin disorders in children. Have each student submit one question for the speaker in advance related to the home management of skin disorders in children.
3. Present a vignette of an adolescent with severe acne. Ask students to discuss:
   (a) current theories about the etiology,
   (b) traditional and new methods of management,
   (c) body image issues related to acne, and
   (d) the nurse's role in caring for this adolescent.
4. Show one of the recommended audio-visual programs on burn injuries and discuss the issues it raises for the child and the parents.
5. Invite a nurse from a burn center to speak to the class about caring for children with burns. Ask the class to discuss:
   (a) immediate care following the burn injury,
   (b) ongoing care until hospital discharge,
   (c) home care and rehabilitation activities, and
   (d) difficulties in the nurse's role in caring for the child with serious burn injuries.

B. Clinical Activities

1. Arrange for students to follow a nurse in a school or day care center to participate in screening for skin infestations. Ask students to evaluate the problems, effectiveness of the screening techniques, and the nursing management of any disorders identified.
2. Assign students to care for a child with a skin disorder in the acute care or home setting and develop a comprehensive care plan for the child and family.

3. Assign students to develop, implement, and evaluate a teaching plan for a specific skin disorder in a child and family.
4. Assign students to visit a dermatology clinic or dermatology office and observe:
   (a) assessment techniques with children,
   (b) types of management used,
   (c) reactions of children, and
   (d) the nurse's role.
5. Assign students to perform an integumentary assessment on any infant or adolescent they are caring for in the acute care setting to determine and document the presence of any skin lesions.
6. Arrange for students to observe the care of a child with severe burn injuries in the PICU or burn unit. Ask students to identify the principal components of both the physical and psychological care that they observe and reactions of the child, family, and nursing staff to this situation.

ALTERATIONS IN PSYCHOSOCIAL FUNCTION

Chapter Overview

Chapter 22 provides an overview of the principal alterations in psychosocial function that affect infants, children, and adolescents. The chapter opens with a general discussion of psychotherapeutic management in this age group. Specific disorders described are autism, attention deficit hyperactivity disorder, mental retardation, eating disorders, substance abuse, depression and anxiety, recurrent abdominal pain, encopresis, childhood schizophrenia, conversion reaction, child abuse, and failure to thrive. Principles of nursing management are applied to practice in a nursing care plan for the child or adolescent hospitalized with depression.

Learning Objectives

- Describe the various treatment modes and therapeutic strategies used to treat children and adolescents with psychosocial disorders.
- Discuss the characteristic behaviors and the medical and nursing management of children who are autistic.
- Describe the characteristic behaviors of a child with ADHD.
- Discuss the care of mentally retarded children in the hospital and the community.

- Describe feeding disorder of infancy or early childhood and outline nursing management of children with this disorder.
- Discuss the care of children with encopresis.
- Differentiate between anorexia nervosa and bulimia nervosa.
- Discuss the medical and nursing management of adolescents with anorexia nervosa and bulimia nervosa.
- List commonly abused drugs and their effects.
- Describe various clinical manifestations of substance abuse.
- Describe characteristic findings of depression and anxiety in children and adolescents.
- Outline risk factors for suicide in children and adolescents.
- Discuss separation anxiety and school phobia and the nursing management of children with these disorders.
- Describe the clinical manifestations of childhood schizophrenia and conversion reaction.
- Recognize the types of child abuse.
- Discuss the nursing management of children who have been abused.
- Discuss the nurse's role in reporting child abuse.
- Describe Munchausen syndrome by proxy and outline the nursing management of children with this disorder.

Key Terms

adaptive functioning
affect
behavior modification
child sexual abuse
cognitive therapy
emotional abuse
emotional neglect
physical abuse
physical neglect
play therapy
stereotypy

Chapter Outline

Psychotherapeutic Management of Children and Adolescents
   Treatment Modes
      Individual Therapy
      Family Therapy
      Group Therapy
   Therapeutic Strategies
      Play Therapy
      Art Therapy
      Behavior Therapy
      Visualization and Guided Imagery
      Hypnosis
   Nurse's Role
Autistic Disorder
   Clinical Manifestations
   Etiology and Pathophysiology
   Diagnostic Tests and Medical Management
   Nursing Assessment
   Nursing Diagnosis
   Nursing Management
Attention Deficit Disorder and Attention Deficit Hyperactivity Disorder
   Clinical Manifestations
   Etiology and Pathophysiology
   Diagnostic Tests and Medical Management
   Nursing Assessment
   Nursing Diagnosis
   Nursing Management
Mental Retardation
   Clinical Manifestations
   Etiology and Pathophysiology

Diagnostic Tests and Medical Management
   Nursing Assessment
   Nursing Diagnosis
   Nursing Management
Eating and Elimination
   Feeding Disorder of Infancy or early Childhood (Failure to Thrive)
      Nursing Management
   Recurrent Abdominal Pain
      Nursing Management
   Encopresis
      Nursing Management
   Anorexia Nervosa
      Clinical Manifestations
      Etiology and Pathophysiology
      Diagnostic Tests and Medical Management
      Nursing Assessment
      Nursing Diagnosis
      Nursing Management
   Bulimia Nervosa
      Clinical Manifestations
      Etiology and Pathophysiology
      Diagnostic Tests and Medical Management
      Nursing Assessment
      Nursing Diagnosis
      Nursing Management
   Compulsive Overeating and Obesity
      Nursing Management
Substance Abuse
   Clinical Manifestations
   Etiology and Pathophysiology
   Diagnostic Tests and Medical Management
   Nursing Assessment
   Nursing Diagnosis
   Nursing Management
Depression and Anxiety
   Depression
      Clinical Manifestations
      Etiology and Pathophysiology
      Diagnostic Tests and Medical Management
      Nursing Assessment
      Nursing Diagnosis
      Nursing Management
   Suicide
      Nursing Management
   Separation Anxiety and School Phobia
      Nursing Management

Schizophrenia
    Nursing Management
  Conversion Reaction
Child Abuse
    Types of Abuse
    Clinical Manifestations
    Etiology and Pathophysiology
    Diagnostic Tests and Medical Management
    Nursing Assessment
    Nursing Diagnosis
    Nursing Management
  Munchausen Syndrome by Proxy
    Nursing Management

Tables

22-1   *DSM-IV* Diagnostic Criteria for Autistic Disorder

22-2   *DSM-IV* Diagnostic Criteria for Attention Deficit Hyperactivity Disorder

22-3   Severity of Mental Retardation

22-4   Characteristics Associated With Three Common Types of Mental Retardation

22-5   Common Causes of Mental Retardation

22-6   *DSM-IV* Diagnostic Criteria for Mental Retardation

22-7   *DSM-IV* Diagnostic Criteria for Anorexia Nervosa.

22-8   *DSM-IV* Diagnostic Criteria for Bulimia Nervosa,

22-9   Commonly Abused Drugs and Their Effects

22-10 Risk Factors for Depression and Anxiety in Children and Adolescents

22-11 Risk Factors for Suicide in Children and Adolescents

22-12 Risk Factors for Child Abuse and Neglect

22-13 Methods of Physical Abuse in Children

22-14 Physical and Behavioral Manifestations of Sexual Abuse in Children and Adolescents

Audio-Visual Resources

1. *The Psychiatry Learning System—Chapter 15: Disorders of Infancy Childhood, and Adolescence, Part 11*
    Videocassette, 43 minutes
    Source: Health Sciences Consortium

2. *Autism: A World Apart*
    Videocassette, 29 minutes
    Source: Fanlight Productions

3. *David: Portrait of a Retarded Youth*
    Videocassette or 16 mm, 28 minutes
    Source: Filmmaker's Library

4. *Dying to be Thin: Surviving Anorexia and Bulimia*
    Videocassette, 58 minutes
    Source: American Journal of Nursing Co.

5. *The Enigma of Anorexia Nervosa: Part I—Delusion and Discord*
    Videocassette, 18 minutes
    Source: Carle Medical Communications

6. *The Enigma of Anorexia Nervosa: Part 11—Clinical Intervention and Rehabilitation*
    Videocassette, 16 minutes
    Source: Carle Medical Communications

7. *The Enigma of Anorexia Nervosa: Part III—The Battle of the Wills*
    Videocassette, 18 minutes
    Source: Carle Medical Communications

8. *Kids and Drugs: A High Price to Pay*
    Videocassette, 28 minutes
    Source: Films for Humanities and Sciences

9. *Stand Up for Yourself—Peer Pressure and Teens*
    16 mm, 15 minutes
    Source: Churchill Films

10. *Suicide: A Teenage Dilemma*
    Videocassette, 30 minutes
    Source: Human Relations Media

11. *Child Abuse*
    Videocassette with Study Guide, 28 minutes
    Source: American Journal of Nursing Co.

12. *Detection and Treatment of Sexually Abused Children, Part I and Part 11*
    Videocassette (2) with Study Guide, 28 minutes
    Source: American Journal of Nursing Co.

13. *Child Abuse: Physical and Behavioral Indicators*
    Videocassette, 28 minutes
    Source: University of Michigan

14. *A Better Beginning (Failure to Thrive)*
    Videocassette, 38 minutes
    Source: University of Michigan

Potential Problem Areas for Students

1. Because it often coexists with developmental learning disabilities, students may not recognize attention deficit hyperactivity disorder (ADHD) as a separate entity. Presenting the *DSM-IV* criteria for ADHD could help students to make this distinction.

2. Students may view anorexia nervosa, bulimia, and compulsive overeating as completely different conditions. An overhead transparency that identifies commonalities of these eating disorders could help students to understand the similar underlying causes and management strategies.

3. Students may have difficulty dealing with abusive parents in the clinical area. Having a representative of Parents Anonymous address abuse issues from a parental perspective should enhance students understanding and communication.

Activities to Foster Critical Thinking

A. CLASSROOM ACTIVITIES

1. Invite a psychiatric clinical nurse specialist to speak to the class about behavioral and psychiatric disorders in children and adolescents. Focus discussion on this nursing role and strategies of nursing management.

2. Invite a representative of Parents Anonymous to speak to the class regarding the problems of child abuse from a parental perspective. Have each student submit one written question for the speaker in advance.

3. Show one of the recommended audio-visual programs and discuss the issues raised related to:
   (a) children's versus parental rights,
   (b) confidentiality,
   (c) causes and effects associated with development, and
   (d) the role of the nurse.

4. Have students role-play one of the following situations:
   (a) admitting an autistic child to an acute care unit,
   (b) assessing a depressed adolescent or suicidal adolescent,
   (c) assessing an adolescent with an eating disorder, or
   (d) interviewing a parent suspected of child abuse.
   Have the class critique the nurse's role in each case.

B. CLINICAL ACTIVITIES

1. Assign students to care for a child or adolescent with any disorder of psychosocial function and develop a comprehensive care plan for the child and family.

2. Arrange for students to sit in on a group therapy session. Have then identify:
   (a) developmental issues,
   (b) intervention techniques, and
   (c) the nursing role.

3. Assign students to interview a child or adolescent with one of the following problems:
   (a) an eating disorder,
   (b) depression or suicide attempt,
   (c) recurrent abdominal pain, or
   (d) a history of abuse.
   Have students evaluate the child's perspective.

4. Assign students to interview the parents of a child with an alteration in psychosocial function to learn:
   (a) the impact on the family and
   (b) the role of the nurse in providing intervention and support.

CONTENTS

1

Nurse's Role in Care of the Ill and Injured Child: Hospital, Community Settings, and Home

1. **The diagnosis phase of the nursing process is the step that**
   a. Identifies the specific actions a nurse takes to manage a health problem
   b. Describes health promotion and health patterns that nurses can manage
   c. Determines the need to define new goals and action plans
   d. Collects data and performs physical examinations on admission and periodically thereafter

   Answer: b

2. **One of the most important considerations in planning the care for all children within our diverse society is**
   a. Financial status
   b. Cultural background
   c. Educational background
   d. Prior health

   Answer: b

3. **The leading cause of death in the adolescent age group is**
   a. Firearm injuries
   b. Homicides
   c. Suicides
   d. Unintentional injuries

   Answer: d

4. **Home health care services for children with needs for skilled nursing are funded primarily through**
   a. State grants
   b. Private donations
   c. Federal funds
   d. Public assistance

   Answer: c

5. **The legal roles and responsibilities of the nurse are defined through**
   a. Institutional job descriptions
   b. The Nurse Practice Act
   c. ANA Code of Ethics
   d. The nursing process

   Answer: b

6. **The process established by a health care institution to identify, evaluate, and reduce injury to patients, visitors, and staff is called**
   a. Quality assurance
   b. Evaluation
   c. Risk management
   d. Case management

   Answer: c

7. **Self-supporting adolescents under the age of 18 who are not subject to parental control are known as**
   a. Mature minors
   b. Emancipated minors
   c. Wards of the State
   d. Waifs

   Answer: b

8. **Minor children and their parents must be informed of their rights while in a health care institution as a result of the**
   a. Advance Directives
   b. Ethical Decision-Making Act
   c. Patient Advocacy Act
   d. Patient Self-Determination Act

   Answer: d

9. **The decision about which child gets an organ for transplant is regulated by the**
   a. Physician of the donor child
   b. Physician of the recipient child
   c. National Organ Transplant Act
   d. Hospital Ethics Review Committee

   Answer: c

10. **Nursing care provided to help restore children to an optimal rate of health is more likely performed in the following health care setting:**
    a. Rehabilitation center
    b. Hospital clinic
    c. Home
    d. Health maintenance organization

    Answer: a

11. **Provisions for free education are provided to all handicapped children between ages 2 and 21 through the**
    a. Public school system
    b. Education for All Handicapped Children Act
    c. Handicap Council of America
    d. National Disability Act

    Answer: b

12. **Exchanging complete and unbiased information between family members and professionals is a key element of**
    a. Socially sensitive care
    b. Contemporary services
    c. Family-centered care
    d. Developmental services

    Answer: c

13. **The leading cause of death in the United States for infants up to 28 days old is**
    a. Congenital anomalies
    b. SIDS
    c. Maternal complications of pregnancy
    d. Disorders related to low birth weight

    Answer: a

14. **The leading cause of death in the United States for infants 1 to 12 months old is**
    a. Respiratory distress syndrome
    b. Congenital anomalies
    c. SIDS
    d. Injuries

    Answer: c

15. **In many states, nursing is defined as**
    a. The treatment of conditions related to human responses
    b. Nursing diagnosis and treatment of complex medical conditions
    c. Professional collaboration with the physician to treat human conditions
    d. Nursing diagnosis and treatment of human responses to health and illness

    Answer: d

16. **The nurse who is involved in monitoring procedures and outcomes of care, as well as measuring compliance with standards of care, is doing**
    a. Quality assurance
    b. Quality improvement
    c. Risk management
    d. Compliance control

    Answer: a

17. When deviations from expected institutional processes and outcomes are identified through an audit of patient records,
    a. Disciplinary action is taken immediately with the nurses who violated outcomes
    b. Patient and family members are notified in writing of the violation
    c. Opportunities to improve care are explored with all care providers
    d. The physician is called and orders are taken to correct the situation

Answer: c

18. The nurse caring for a 14-year-old boy who refuses medical treatment understands
    a. The boy's parents must be informed immediately
    b. Mature minors can refuse treatment in some states
    c. This response is a normal, expected response to treatment
    d. The treatment must be given regardless of the boy's refusal

Answer: b

19. Jehovah's Witnesses oppose blood transfusions for themselves and their children because they believe
    a. Transfusions are equivalent to the oral intake of blood
    b. After transfusions, they will take on characteristics of the blood donor
    c. The blood is contaminated
    d. The process used to obtain the blood is immoral

Answer: a

20. The nurse suspects that the 4-year-old boy she has been caring for has been abused by his parents. The nurse must
    a. Observe parent/child interactions at all times
    b. Recognize this as a normal response to parental stress
    c. Report the suspected abuse to the appropriate agency
    d. Get a doctor's order to restrict the parents from seeing the child

Answer: c

21. Comprehensive interdisciplinary plans for a specific condition that describe the sequence and timing of interventions are called
    a. Critical pathways
    b. Physician plans of care
    c. Treatment continuums
    d. Nursing care plans

Answer: a

22. Professional Practice Standards for Pediatric Nursing Practice include all of the following, except
    a. Collecting health data
    b. Auditing health records
    c. Analyzing assessment data to determine diagnosis
    d. Implementing interventions identified on care plan

Answer: b

23. In the event of an emergency need for surgery to save the life of a child, informed consent
    a. Does not have to be obtained
    b. Can be obtained from a sibling
    c. Must be obtained from both parents
    d. Can only be authorized by the hospital chaplain

Answer: a

24. A 14-year-old girl, who has just found out she is pregnant, pleads with the nurse not to tell her parents. The nurse must
    a. Report the condition to the public health department
    b. Inform the child's parents immediately
    c. Recognize that mature minors can receive treatment without informing parents
    d. Inform the child's school nurse of the condition

Answer: c

2

GROWTH AND DEVELOPMENT

1. The process of developing from the head downward through the body and toward the feet is termed
   a. Cephalodistal
   b. Cephalocaudal
   c. Proximodistal
   d. Proximocaudal

   Answer: b

2. The process by which development proceeds from the center of the body outward to the extremities is termed
   a. Cephalodistal
   b. Cephalocaudal
   c. Proximodistal
   d. Proximocaudal

   Answer: c

3. When caring for a toddler in Erikson's stage of autonomy versus shamed doubt, it is important for the nurse to recognize
   a. The need to toilet train the child
   b. That independence should be encouraged in activities of daily living
   c. That the child needs to be held often
   d. The need to name objects for the child and describe their function

   Answer: b

4. In working with school-age children, the nurse who knocks on the child's door before entering the room and who encourages the child to engage in favorite activities is applying the theories of
   a. Erikson and Piaget
   b. Piaget and Kohlberg
   c. Freud and Piaget
   d. Freud and Erikson

   Answer: d

5. The nurse is applying Piaget's preoperational stage of cognitive development to interventions when
   a. Involving parents in care
   b. Planning playtime for the child
   c. Explaining all procedures and treatments
   d. Encouraging the child to initiate play activities

   Answer: c

6. The nurse presents a plan of care to a teenager to consider, understanding that, during Kohlberg's postconventional stage of moral development, the teenager
   a. Is capable of making decisions after considering differing moral approaches
   b. Makes a decision based on a desire to please others
   c. Espouses only one moral point of view
   d. Expects to be autonomous

   Answer: a

7. The nurse who uses positive reinforcement immediately upon teaching a child the importance of daily hygiene is applying
   a. Social learning theory
   b. Behaviorism
   c. Temperament theory
   d. Bandurism

Answer: b

8. A mother asks you when her newborn's "soft spots" will disappear. You explain that the anterior fontanel "closes" during the second year of life and the posterior fontanel closes between
   a. 2 and 4 months of age
   b. 5 and 6 months of age
   c. 12 and 18 months of age
   d. 2 and 3 years of age

Answer: a

9. A 3-month-old will grasp a rattle that is placed in her hand. Her mother asks when she will be able to grasp a rattle without help. You answer that fine motor ability develops by
   a. 4 to 6 months
   b. 5 to 7 months
   c. 6 to 8 months
   d. 7 to 9 months

Answer: a

10. A 6-month-old sits alone momentarily. His father asks you when he will be able to sit alone for sustained periods of time. You explain that gross motor ability is usually present by
    a. 6 months
    b. 7 months
    c. 8 months
    d. 9 months

Answer: c

11. A mother asks you when her 8-month-old will be able to eat with a spoon. You explain that, in general, infants begin attempts at feeding themselves between
    a. 8 and 10 months
    b. 10 and 12 months
    c. 14 and 16 months
    d. 18 and 24 months

Answer: b

12. In teaching parents to avoid putting the child to bed with a bottle of milk or juice, you explain the significance of
    a. Nursing bottle syndrome
    b. Bottle dependency syndrome
    c. Otitis externa
    d. Suddent infant death syndrome

Answer: a

13. While teaching parents about appropriate finger foods for their 1-year-old, the nurse cautions against foods which commonly cause choking, such as
    a. Pieces of turkey and beef
    b. Cooked carrots and beans
    c. Cheerios and toast
    d. Hot dogs and grapes

Answer: d

14. Activities that the nurse can expect to assess in a toddler include
    a. Building a tower of four blocks, undressing self, and drawing a circle
    b. Dressing and undressing self, jumping, running, and kicking a ball
    c. Pouring liquids, throwing a ball overhand, and drawing circles
    d. Walking up and down stairs, pushing and pulling toys, and kicking a ball

Answer: a

15. In discussing toilet training with the mother of an 18-month-old, the nurse describes the signs of readiness in the child, which include
    a. Regressive behavior during toilet training
    b. Walking around by holding onto furniture
    c. Wetting the diaper every hour
    d. The ability to pull pants up and down

Answer: d

16. It is important to allow toddlers to make choices from a variety of foods and provide opportunities for self-feeding because they
    a. Are trying to imitate behaviors
    b. Need to reinforce their autonomy
    c. Will have a temper tantrum otherwise
    d. Will become negative in behavior

Answer: b

17. In teaching injury prevention to the parents of a toddler, the nurse advises parents to lock up all medications and poisonous materials because the child
    a. Is now tall enough to reach these cupboards
    b. Is in the stage of autonomy
    c. Can climb onto chairs and up ladders
    d. Can solve puzzles

Answer: c

18. In planning for therapeutic play for a preschooler, the nurse recognizes that preschoolers are generally involved in
    a. Dramatic play
    b. Imitative play
    c. Independent play
    d. Gang play

Answer: a

19. There is a social dimension to the play of preschoolers, termed associative play. During this type of play, children
    a. Act out fantasies
    b. Interact when doing a project
    c. Use increasing manual dexterity
    d. Engage in more complex manipulation

Answer: b

20. Teaching a child about certain procedures and treatments is best accomplished
    a. In small groups
    b. At mealtimes
    c. Through play activities
    d. With the help of a psychologist

Answer: c

21. In teaching parents about safety, the nurse explains that, although laws vary from state to state, a child car seat should be used until the child
    a. Weighs 40 pounds and is 40 inches tall
    b. Is 5 years of age
    c. Goes to school
    d. Weighs 18 pounds and is 100 inches tall

Answer: a

22. School-age children, according to Erikson, are in the stage of industry. In caring for these children, the nurse facilitates a sense of achievement in their activities to develop
    a. Trust
    b. Self-esteem
    c. Autonomy
    d. Transductive reasoning

Answer: b

23. The school-age child understands an incision will heal and that his arm will return to normal once the intravenous needle is removed because he has learned the concept of
    a. Centration
    b. Conservation
    c. Concretism
    d. Transducive reasoning

Answer: b

24. In teaching school-age children, it is important to use pictures to reinforce verbal descriptions because these children are in the cognitive stage of
    a. Preoperational thought
    b. Conventional thought
    c. Concrete operational thought
    d. Sensorimotor thought

Answer: c

25. When discussing injury prevention with adolescents, the nurse should remember that
    a. Teens rely on concrete experiences
    b. Teens understand various roles
    c. Adolescents think no harm can come to them
    d. Adolescents like to engage in solitary activities

Answer: c

3

PEDIATRIC ASSESSMENT

1. **To determine if a dark-skinned child has either jaundice or cyanosis, the nurse should**
   a. Examine the skin in sunlight
   b. Inspect the entire skin surface
   c. Blanch the gums by pressing them lightly for 1 to 2 seconds
   d. Inspect the pupils

   Answer: c

2. **The nurse pinches a small amount of skin on the child's abdomen to assess skin**
   a. Temperature
   b. Capillary refill
   c. Moistness
   d. Turgor

   Answer: d

3. **When assessing skin lesions, the nurse describes the following as secondary lesions:**
   a. Scars, ulcers, and fissures
   b. Macules, papules, and fissures
   c. Nodules, tumors, and wheals
   d. Vesicles, pustules, and bullae

   Answer: a

4. **Upon palpation of the infant's head, the fontanels should feel**
   a. Tense and bulging
   b. Soft and sunken
   c. Flat and firm
   d. Flat and tense

   Answer: c

5. **When a bright light is shone into one eye, the normal response is**
   a. Constriction of the exposed pupil
   b. Constriction of both pupils
   c. Dilation of the exposed pupil
   d. Dilation of both pupils

   Answer: b

6. **A foul-smelling, purulent discharge in the external auditory canal or nostrils may indicate**
   a. The presence of a sinus infection
   b. Mastoiditis
   c. The presence of a foreign body
   d. An inner ear infection

   Answer: c

7. **Initial screening for hearing loss in infants and toddlers involves**
   a. Clapping the hands at various levels of loudness
   b. Whispering softly
   c. Using a tuning fork
   d. Using noise makers with different frequencies

   Answer: d

8. **Parents notice a white coating on their infant's tongue, which the nurse assesses as**
   a. Thrush
   b. Overfeeding syndrome
   c. Dehydration
   d. Geographic tongue

   Answer: a

9. **In examing a 2-year-old, you palpate firm, clearly defined, nontender movable cervical lymph nodes 1 cm in diameter. This finding**
   a. Indicates that a throat infection is present
   b. Indicates that an ear infection is present
   c. Is lymphadenopathy
   d. Is normal

   Answer: d

10. **The best auscultation sites to identify absent or diminished breath sounds in infants and young children are**
    a. Apex and midaxillary areas
    b. Intercostal spaces
    c. Midclavicular areas
    d. Above the diaphragm

    Answer: a

11. **In assessing abnormal breath sounds, the nurse notes the location, the respiratory phase, and**
    a. The quality of the voice
    b. The transmission of voice sounds
    c. Changes in sound when the child coughs or shifts position
    d. Any hoarseness or stridor when assessing for tactile fremitus

    Answer: c

12. **Gynecomastia in adolescent males**
    a. Can be a normal finding
    b. Is always normal
    c. Indicates that they will cross dress
    d. Indicates adrenogenital syndrome

    Answer: a

13. **You have auscultated an infant's heart rate for a minute and note a sinus arrhythmia. This finding**
    a. Should be reevaluated after changing the infant's position
    b. Is abnormal
    c. Is normal
    d. Is indicative of heart disease

    Answer: c

14. **Cyanosis is most commonly associated with**
    a. Asthma
    b. Respiratory infections
    c. Pneumonia
    d. Congenital heart defects

    Answer: d

15. **In the newborn, continued drainage from the umbilicus after the umbilical stump falls off**
    a. May indicate an infection or a granuloma
    b. Is normal for several days
    c. Is associated with an umbilical hernia
    d. Is associated with separation of the rectus abdominis muscle

    Answer: a

16. **When examining the scrotum of adolescent boys, the nurse**
    a. Avoids palpation
    b. Assesses the cremasteric reflex as indicative of undescended testicles
    c. Notes scrotal rugae as abnormal
    d. Ensures that the inguinal canals are blocked off before palpating the testes

    Answer: d

17. While assessing a 2-week-old male, the nurse notes that one side of the scrotum is enlarged and firm and cannot be pushed through the external inguinal ring. This finding is indicative of
    a. An inguinal hernia
    b. A hydrocele or incarcerated hernia
    c. Cremasteric reflex
    d. A blocked spermatic duct
    Answer: b

18. Extra skin folds and a larger circumference in one extremity when compared to the other may indicate
    a. A shorter extremity
    b. Dislocation of the hip
    c. Differences in alignment
    d. A flexed extremity
    Answer: a

19. The nurse is assessing a 7-year-old girl's joints and notes swelling, warmth, and tenderness of the joints. This finding may be indicative of
    a. Hyptertonia
    b. Muscle atrophy
    c. Juvenile rheumatoid arthritis
    d. Muscular dystrophy
    Answer: c

20. The nurse assesses a lateral curvature of the spine in a 10-year-old boy. This finding is indicative of
    a. Scoliosis
    b. Lordosis
    c. Kyphosis
    d. Allis' sign
    Answer: a

21. While assessing a 2-month-old infant, you startle the infant suddenly to elicit the
    a. Palmer reflex
    b. Moro reflex
    c. Placing reflex
    d. Babinski reflex
    Answer: b

22. In assessing height and weight of a child against the age-appropriate standardized growth curves, the nurse notes a measurement below the 10th percentile. This finding may be indicative of
    a. Undernutrition
    b. Overnutrition
    c. Neurological dysfunction
    d. Adequate growth and development
    Answer: a

23. An enlarged thyroid in a child may be indicative of the following nutrient deficiency:
    a. Protein
    b. Minerals
    c. Calories
    d. Vitamins
    Answer: b

24. Dry, scaling lips, poor tooth development, and bleeding gums may be indicative of the following nutrient deficiency:
    a. Vitamins
    b. Minerals
    c. Proteins
    d. Fats
    Answer: a

25. Checking a 3-year-old child's feet for the presence of an arch is best done with the child
    a. Lying in a prone position
    b. Standing erect
    c. Standing on tiptoe
    d. Lying in a supine position
    Answer: c

4

Nursing Considerations for the Hospitalized Child

1. **A 3-year-old child who has been in the hospital for 5 days no longer cries when his parents leave and cries when his parents reappear. These behaviors may indicate**
   a. A healthy and adaptive response
   b. Despair and denial
   c. Low self-esteem
   d. Suspected child abuse

   Answer: b

2. **Considering the developmental aspects of adolescence, what is a nursing diagnosis which may be most appropriate for a teenager hospitalized for chemotherapy?**
   a. High risk for disuse phenomenon
   b. Self-care deficit
   c. Sensory-perceptual alteration
   d. Body image disturbance

   Answer: d

3. **Anxiety and fear of procedures and treatments in an adolescent can be reduced significantly if the nurse**
   a. Plans a hospital tour with the adolescent and parents
   b. Encourages the adolescent to go to a health fair
   c. Teaches stress management techniques
   d. Gives the adolescent information to read

   Answer: c

4. **In discussing the purpose of sending a child to a rehabilitation unit, the nurse explains to the parents that the primary objective of rehabilitation is**
   a. To assess the individual child and determine developmental needs
   b. To teach parents how to help their child to master developmental milestones
   c. To assist parent and child in the adaptation process
   d. To help the child reach his or her maximum potential and achievement of skills

   Answer: d

5. **In preparing a teaching plan for a child with hearing deficits, the nurse recognizes that the most effective learning strategies to incorporate are**
   a. Shorter teaching sessions and audiovisual equipment
   b. Visual and tactile presentations
   c. Small group sessions and computer resources
   d. Frequent reinforcement and written materials

   Answer: b

6. One of the primary objectives of Child Life Programs in the hospital setting is to
   a. Teach parents effective discipline techniques
   b. Offer activities to facilitate play and stress reduction
   c. Encourage use of car seats and safety belts
   d. Promote the child's understanding of the body and its functions

Answer: b

7. The Goodenough Draw-A-Person Test is a diagnostic tool used to assess a child's
   a. Psychomotor ability
   b. Relationship with parents
   c. Artistic ability
   d. Cognitive level

Answer: d

8. In trying to determine a child's knowledge of his/her own body, the nurse may use the following tool:
   a. The Gellert Index
   b. The Denver Scale
   c. Beck's Inventory
   d. The Rahe and Holmes Scale

Answer: a

9. The nurse promotes a sense of stability in a toddler who is restrained in the hospital by
   a. Turning out the lights and allowing the child rest time
   b. Reading familiar stories to the child
   c. Playing cartoons during hours awake
   d. Placing the child in a room with another toddler

Answer: b

10. The nurse can alleviate many fears and fantasies of bodily harm in a preschool child with the use of
    a. Stress management techniques
    b. Picture books
    c. Therapeutic play with a doll
    d. Videotapes

Answer: c

11. When working with the teenage patient population, the nurse considers the following therapeutic recreation in meeting developmental needs:
    a. Interactions with other adolescents at social activities
    b. Interactive computer video games
    c. Working with puzzles
    d. Bookmobile visits

Answer: a

12. In preparing a toddler for a procedure such as a blood draw, the nurse should explain the procedure
    a. Just prior to the procedure
    b. Only to the parents
    c. Using picture books
    d. Several times in advance of the procedure

Answer: a

13. When performing an invasive procedure on an infant, the nurse encourages parents to
    a. Leave the unit so they don't hear the crying
    b. Hold the infant following the procedure
    c. Restrain the infant so the procedure can be performed quickly
    d. Allow the infant to cry after the procedure

Answer: b

14. In working with a school-aged child, acceptance of procedures may be promoted by
    a. Giving an in-depth explanation of what to expect
    b. Presenting a graphic video of the procedure
    c. Proceeding through the procedure without discussing it
    d. Offering a choice of reward upon completion of the procedure

Answer: d

15. Procedures performed on young children are usually done in the treatment room because
    a. It is the most aseptic environment for the treatment
    b. Children are less afraid in a different environment
    c. The child's room is considered a safe haven
    d. The treatment room is soundproof

Answer: c

16. **When parents of a chronically ill child are managing their child's health care at home, the nurse can assist them in meeting their psychosocial needs by**
    a. Arranging for meals to be brought in
    b. Encouraging options for respite
    c. Arranging for private pay home care coverage
    d. Insisting that the child be placed in a long-term care facility

    Answer: b

17. **When planning for the ongoing needs of a hospitalized child, discharge planning begins**
    a. When the physician writes an order for discharge planning
    b. As early as possible in the hospitalization
    c. When it has been determined that parents cannot provide the care
    d. When all community resources have been notified

    Answer: b

18. **The parents of a 7-year-old hospitalized with a fractured femur are concerned over the acting-out behavior of their 5-year-old daughter. The nurse explains that**
    a. The 5-year-old may be emotionally traumatized by the event
    b. This behavior may be indicative of antisocial tendencies
    c. This is not normal and the 5-year-old should be evaluated by a psychologist
    d. Siblings often feel jealous when the ill brother or sister monopolizes the parents' time

    Answer: d

19. **The practice of allowing parents to stay in the hospitalized child's room to assist in caring for the child is called**
    a. Case managing
    b. Rooming in
    c. Participatory care
    d. The 1 + 1 plan

    Answer: b

20. **The mother of a 4-year-old girl is concerned because her daughter insists that her teddy bear made her sick by magic. The nurse explains that**
    a. The child should be corrected immediately and given another explanation
    b. It is common for preschoolers to think an unrelated event has caused their illness
    c. The child is suffering from delusions and should be evaluated by a psychiatrist
    d. Stuffed animals can cause certain types of illness in children

    Answer: b

21. **When a hospitalized child begins to demonstrate regressive behaviors, the nurse recognizes**
    a. Parents may be too involved in the care
    b. The need to restrain the child from such behaviors
    c. That this is a normal response to stress
    d. The child may have deep emotional problems

    Answer: c

22. **In preparing an explanation of a surgical procedure for a preschool patient, the nurse offers that the surgery**
    a. Has many risks involved
    b. Will be performed after the child goes to sleep
    c. May be painful, but analgesics will be provided
    d. Will fix the child's body

    Answer: d

23. **An appropriate expected outcome for the diagnosis of Risk for Complication Related to Surgical Procedure and Anesthetic is that the child will have a bowel movement within**
    a. 24 hours after surgery
    b. 36 hours after surgery
    c. 2 to 3 days after surgery
    d. 4 to 6 days after surgery

    Answer: c

24. **An effective nursing intervention to promote return to normal bowel function following a surgical procedure is**
   a. Increased activity as ordered and tolerated
   b. Encouraging oral fluids if bowel sounds are absent
   c. Coughing and deep breathing
   d. Restricting all food until after the first bowel movement

Answer: a

25. **To assist in achieving pain control following surgery in a child, the nurse recognizes the importance of**
   a. Limiting the frequency of medication to discourage dependency
   b. Using primarily nonpharmacologic interventions to control pain
   c. Administering prescribed pain medication on a regular basis
   d. Allowing parents to make the decision regarding how often to medicate for pain

Answer: c

5

Nursing Considerations for the Child in the Community

1. **Managed care organizations advocate for newborn discharge 24 to 48 hours after birth primarily to**
   a. Facilitate infant-parent bonding
   b. Protect the infant from nosocomial infections
   c. Reduce health care costs
   d. Market home care services
   Answer: c

2. **The primary reason schools must provide education to all disabled children, regardless of health status, is because they are**
   a. Morally and ethically obligated to provide education to all children
   b. Mandated by federal law to provide education to all disabled children
   c. Prepared to care for ill children
   d. Providing opportunities for all children to learn about disabilities
   Answer: b

3. **The nurse working with children in the community recognizes a medical home as a**
   a. Happy and harmonious family unit
   b. Home in which children are safe from household injury
   c. Long-term rehabilitation center for children
   d. Regular source of primary health care
   Answer: d

4. **The nurse explains the importance of health supervision to new parents as**
   a. Periodic health care screenings during the first 5 years of life
   b. Services which focus on disease and injury prevention and health promotion during childhood
   c. A care provider service for assisting parents to find transportation to the child's appointments
   d. Promotion of healthy lifestyles and health practices among children
   Answer: b

5. **Screening tests which provide the most accurate results have**
   a. High sensitivity and low specificity
   b. Low sensititivity and high specificity
   c. High sensitivity and high specificity
   d. Low sensitivity and low specificity
   Answer: c

6. **Young children living in homes built prior to 1960 are at greatest risk for**
   a. Inhalation of toxic fumes from furnace
   b. Lead poisoning
   c. Respiratory distress from old carpet fibers
   d. Termite bites and subsequent infection
   Answer: b

7. **When administering a developmental surveillance exam, the nurse is assessing**
   a. Parenting behaviors of child's parent
   b. Fine and gross motor skills, language, and psychosocial behavior
   c. Task resolution across the developmental years
   d. The child's development against the norm

   Answer: b

8. **An organization to which the nurse may refer families who want to learn about injury prevention strategies is**
   a. WIC
   b. SAFE KIDS
   c. SAFCO
   d. DARE

   Answer: b

9. **The nurse working with school-aged children between 5 and 12 recognizes the focus on health education centers around**
   a. Teaching personal care and hygiene
   b. Eating disorders
   c. Drug and alcohol use
   d. Sexual activity

   Answer: a

10. **The definition of a child with special health care needs is the child who**
    a. Has an acute condition requiring special treatment
    b. Has a chronic condition of 3 months' or greater duration
    c. Is identified by the school nurse as "gifted"
    d. Depends upon technological equipment to learn

    Answer: b

11. **In teaching children with asthma and their parents about taking medication, the nurse stresses taking prn medications**
    a. Sparingly
    b. Only after symptoms become evident
    c. In response to changes indicated by the peak flow meter
    d. In the evening hours due to sedative effects

    Answer: c

12. **Which of the following nursing diagnoses addresses the impact that asthma has on a child's developing self-esteem?**
    a. Ineffective management of therapeutic regime
    b. Body image disturbance
    c. Anxiety
    d. Role conflict

    Answer: b

13. **In planning a vision screening test, the school nurse invites the following to participate:**
    a. Children with known visual problems
    b. All children whose parents wear glasses
    c. All children in the school
    d. Only children who demonstrate difficulty learning

    Answer: c

14. **To ensure that the health care needs of children with chronic conditions are met, the school nurse refers to**
    a. The State Code for Nursing
    b. Public health standards and protocols
    c. An individual school health plan
    d. The collaborative health record

    Answer: c

15. **When a child with chronic health problems requires medical treatment during school hours, it is essential that**
    a. A physician's written instructions for care be followed
    b. One of the parents provides the care
    c. The child be accompanied by a home care nurse
    d. The child be separated from other children

    Answer: a

16. **When working with the family of a child with a chronic condition, the nurse observes ineffective coping skills and recognizes that**
    a. The family is demonstrating resilience
    b. Nursing support is needed
    c. This is unnatural and dysfunctional
    d. The family unit is breaking up

    Answer: b

17. The Family APGAR screening tool focuses on the family's
    a. Anger, problems, grieving, alienation, and repression
    b. Attitude, pride, gratitude, acceptance, and resources
    c. Adaptation, partnership, growth, affection, and resolve
    d. Agility, patience, generosity, affect, and reality

Answer: c

18. A visit to the home by the school nurse when all family members are present is indicated when the
    a. School suspects abusive behavior
    b. Nurse utilizes the HOME tool
    c. Family is unable to come into the school
    d. Family is reported to be under caregiver role strain

Answer: b

19. In establishing a therapeutic relationship with the family of a child with a chronic illness, the nurse builds resiliency by
    a. Anticipating all concerns and addressing them
    b. Providing all answers to the family's questions
    c. Asking questions to direct the family's thinking
    d. Referring the family to social services for counseling

Answer: c

20. Children who require skilled nursing care to support vital functions are referred to as
    a. Acutely ill
    b. Medically fragile
    c. Dependent
    d. Incapacitated

Answer: b

21. A screening test value stated as the percentage of children testing positive for a condition when they truly have that condition is referred to as
    a. Disability
    b. Specificity
    c. Sensitivity
    d. Health index

Answer: c

22. A screening test value stated as the percentage of children testing negative for a condition who do not have the condition is referred to as
    a. Specificity
    b. Sensitivity
    c. Health index
    d. Margin of error

Answer: a

23. Procedures used by the community health nurse to detect the presence of a health condition before symptoms are apparent are called
    a. Immunizations
    b. Screening tests
    c. Research studies
    d. Developmental surveillance

Answer: b

24. A health care condition is considered chronic if it lasts
    a. 4 weeks
    b. 5 weeks
    c. 2 months
    d. 3 months

Answer: d

25. When the community health nurse provides anticipatory guidance, the nurse focuses on
    a. What to expect during the child's current and next stage of development
    b. Preparing parents for the financial obligations anticipated with hospitalization
    c. Teaching parenting skills
    d. Potential problems anticipated in caring for a child with a chronic condition

Answer: a

6

THE CHILD WITH A
LIFE-THREATENING ILLNESS OR INJURY

1. **Billy screams whenever a nurse approaches his crib. In which age group is stranger anxiety most evident?**
   a. 1 to 6 months
   b. 6 to 12 months
   c. 12 to 15 months
   d. 15 to 18 months

   Answer: b

2. **Among the four most significant stressors for hospitalized children in all age groups is**
   a. Fear of bodily injury
   b. Fear of the dark
   c. Stranger anxiety
   d. Separation from peer group

   Answer: a

3. **What is the most appropriate nursing diagnosis for the 10-year-old who was admitted to the PICU 48 hours ago for the treatment of status asthmaticus?**
   a. Impaired physical mobility related to trauma, pain, or the use of physical restraints
   b. Diversional activity deficit related to the monotony of confinement
   c. Sleep pattern disturbance related to medications, pain, fear, or critical care environment
   d. Self-esteem disturbance related to the loss of body function, hospitalization, or loss of independence and autonomy

   Answer: c

4. **When a child is either in a PICU or has a life-threatening illness, the situation often becomes a crisis for the family because**
   a. It is more difficult to provide psychosocial support
   b. The usual coping methods are not effective
   c. The environment is impersonal
   d. The family has lack of trust in health care providers

   Answer: b

5. **Once a child has been admitted to a PICU, it is important to develop interventions that focus on the needs of family members and to keep them informed about the child's status to**
   a. Ease their discomfort in this high-tech setting
   b. Demonstrate concern for the welfare of individual family members
   c. Help them adjust more readily to the crisis situation
   d. Evaluate the ability of family members to manage the crisis

   Answer: c

6. In dealing with the stress of having a child in the PICU, the parents of a 5-year-old boy express themselves inappropriately to the staff. The nurse recognizes that the child will most likely
   a. Apologize for his parents' behaviors
   b. Become very quiet with the staff
   c. Mirror the parents' behaviors and responses
   d. Be cheerful and well behaved

Answer: c

7. In a crisis situation, parents may lose trust in the hospital staff when
   a. The course of an illness is given to them
   b. Information is withheld from them
   c. Unforeseen complications develop
   d. Updates are not given consistently

Answer: b

8. The nurse in a PICU encourages parents to stay in this critical care environment because their presence
   a. Serves to comfort their child
   b. Relieves the nurse of providing physical care
   c. Makes them available to answer questions
   d. Facilitates the teaching that needs to be done

Answer: a

9. Considering the intensity of parental experiences when a child is critically ill, what is the most important aspect of communications with parents among nursing staff?
   a. Availability of information
   b. Consistency of information
   c. Information presented in a concise, professional manner
   d. Sparing parents the details of care

Answer: b

10. When the parent of a child in the PICU asks a nurse, "What should I tell his brother?", the nurse should reply that it is essential for a healthy sibling to be
    a. Informed in a language appropriate to his age and developmental level
    b. Protected as much as possible
    c. Told just a little bit of what a parent knows
    d. Informed of his brother's positive progress only

Answer: a

11. Parents of a child who has died in the PICU ask if they can hold their son. How should his primary nurse respond to this request?
    a. Get an order from the physician
    b. Deny it to protect them from additional pain
    c. Allow them the privacy to hold their son
    d. Tell them it would be better to leave

Answer: c

12. In assisting a family to discuss the death of their son with their 4-year-old daughter, the nurse stresses the fact that a preschooler's understanding of death is based upon the belief that death is
    a. Permanent
    b. Reversible
    c. Make-believe
    d. A spiritual event

Answer: b

13. The parents of a 4-year-old with a chronic illness are concerned that their child does not understand how ill he really is. The nurse explains that a child generally cannot comprehend the seriousness of an illness until the age of
    a. 3 years
    b. 5 years
    c. 7 years
    d. 9 years

Answer: b

14. Nurses working with children in the PICU can promote comfort and security for the child when parents are not available by
    a. Dimming the lights and playing soft music
    b. Discussing his or her fears with the child
    c. Providing the child with his or her favorite toys or blankets
    d. Turning off the alarms on the monitoring equipment

Answer: c

15. **A common coping strategy that nurses often use when caring for a dying child and his or her family is to**
    a. Spend more time with the child and family
    b. Become overprotective toward the child and family
    c. Verbalize their frustrations in dealing with the child and family
    d. Distance themselves socially from the child and family

Answer: d

16. **An appropriate outcome for the diagnosis of powerlessness related to inability to communicate, and the lack of privacy and control, is that the child will**
    a. Express satisfaction over increased sense of control
    b. Report increased self-esteem
    c. Demonstrate less anxiety
    d. Verbalize effective coping strategies

Answer: a

17. **The nurse encourages the parents of an unconscious child to talk and comfort the child because**
    a. This will alleviate the parents' feelings of guilt
    b. Someone must stay with the child at all times
    c. The child may still hear their voices and feel their touch
    d. The parents will be able to alert the staff when the child awakes

Answer: c

18. **To promote a sense of bodily control in a child who has a serious illness, the nurse should**
    a. Allow the child to make all decisions about care
    b. Offer choices whenever possible related to physical care
    c. Encourage the child to trust the nursing staff
    d. Anticipate the child's needs and respond to them

Answer: b

19. **The parents of a 7-year-old boy, who has just been sent to surgery for repair of serious injuries as a result of an automobile accident, repeatedly ask questions of the staff. The nurse explains to the staff that the parents**
    a. Have many emotional problems
    b. Are showing behavior that is highly suspicious and bears close observation
    c. Are expressing guilt over their role in the accident
    d. Are experiencing shock and disbelief related to the crisis

Answer: d

20. **The typical response of parents who have relinquished their parental role of caring for their child to the hospital staff is a feeling of**
    a. Relief
    b. Anger
    c. Loss
    d. Uncertainty

Answer: c

21. **The stage which parents experience as their child recovers, improves, and prepares for discharge is termed the**
    a. Readjustment stage
    b. Grieving stage
    c. Termination stage
    d. Anticipatory stage

Answer: a

22. **Nurses can offer psychological support to the parents of critically ill children most appropriately by**
    a. Providing information as requested
    b. Helping them to focus on the positive aspects of their child
    c. Ordering meals for them
    d. Allowing them to make unlimited phone calls

Answer: b

23. The preoccupation with illness, fears, and anxiety over the changes in normal body function and appearance that a dying child expresses is referred to as
   a. Death watch
   b. Death anxiety
   c. Acceptance
   d. Denial

Answer: b

24. The mother of a 3-year-old just diagnosed with *Haemophilus influenzae* repeatedly states, "If only I took her in to see the doctor earlier...." The nurse recognizes this response as
   a. Guilt
   b. Anger
   c. Ambivalence
   d. Denial

Answer: a

25. After the death of a child, the parents may request some time alone with the body. The nurse allows the parents
   a. To spend not more than 10 minutes at the bedside
   b. 1 hour to be with their child
   c. As much time as they need to say goodbye
   d. To discuss their concerns with the chaplain

Answer: c

7

PAIN ASSESSMENT AND MANAGEMENT

1. **In the past, pain medication for children was ordered only as needed, if at all, because of the belief that**
   a. Children did not feel the same intensity of pain as adults
   b. The danger of respiratory depression caused by narcotics was too great
   c. Pain was too complex for children to understand
   d. The usual pain medications were far too strong for children

   Answer: a

2. **At what age can children demonstrate the anticipatory fear of pain?**
   a. 3 months
   b. 6 months
   c. 9 months
   d. 12 months

   Answer: b

3. **Recent research indicates that the following pediatric age group is the most sensitive to pain:**
   a. Premature infants
   b. Full-term infants
   c. 6 to 9 months
   d. 5 to 6 years

   Answer: a

4. **In preparing pain medication for a 10-year-old boy, the nurse administers acetaminophen along with an opioid analgesic because**
   a. The nurse anticipates a rise in temperature with the pain
   b. The effectiveness of the narcotic will be increased
   c. Acetaminophen will decrease the resultant gastric discomfort from the narcotic
   d. The combination of the two drugs will induce sleep

   Answer: b

5. **The nurse caring for a 5-year-old girl in acute pain may elect to administer IV pain medication as opposed to giving her an injection because**
   a. An injection will take longer to work
   b. The child may not have enough muscle tissue to give the injection
   c. Preschoolers relate pain to injury and the injection would cause more pain
   d. An injection offers less pain relef than pain medication given by IV

   Answer: c

6. In trying to determine the level of intensity of pain in a 9-year-old child, the most appropriate pain assessment scale to use is the
   a. Eland Color Tool
   b. Oucher Scale
   c. CHEOPS Tool
   d. NIPS Scale

Answer: a

7. The numeric pain intensity scale which is typically used in the adult setting can be used with pediatric patients once they reach the age of
   a. 6
   b. 7
   c. 8
   d. 9

Answer: d

8. Administration of opioids by the oral route is as effective as by IM and IV routes when the drug is given
   a. With milk
   b. In lesser amounts
   c. In an equianalgesic dose
   d. Along with an antiemetic

Answer: c

9. The nurse who has just administered an opioid analgesic must be aware of the following common side effects to monitor:
   a. Sedation, nausea, vomiting, constipation, and itching
   b. Gastrointestinal pain, diarrhea, and vomiting
   c. Facial flushing, muscle weakness, and spasms
   d. Bradycardia, seizure activity, and headaches

Answer: a

10. When administering opioids to a child in an unstable condition, the nurse must make the following assessment prior to determining the correct prn dose:
    a. Neurological status
    b. Cardiorespiratory status
    c. The child's preference for taking PO, IM, and IV medication
    d. Intake and output

Answer: b

11. Nonsteroidal anti-inflammatory drugs are most commonly used for
    a. Children who have allergies to aspirin
    b. Intense, acute episodes of pain
    c. Bone, inflammatory, and rheumatoid conditions
    d. Cutaneous pain

Answer: c

12. Which one of the following NSAIDs has less of a peripheral anti-inflammatory effect?
    a. Acetaminophen
    b. Ibuprofen
    c. Tolmetin
    d. Choline magnesium trisalicylate

Answer: a

13. Patient-controlled analgesia (PCA) is prescribed for children who are old enough to
    a. Understand the mechanisms involved in the pump system
    b. Understand that pushing the button will give them pain relief
    c. Verbalize the potential side effects of the medication
    d. Count the number of times they push the button each hour

Answer: b

14. When pain medication is administered through the epidural route, the nurse recognizes that
    a. Larger quantities of the drug are infused
    b. There is a greater chance for sleep pattern disturbance
    c. The catheter needs to be changed every 8 hours to avoid infection
    d. Only minute doses of the drug are actually being given

Answer: d

15. When a child has been getting regular doses of codeine, the most common GI side effect the nurse can expect is
    a. Constipation
    b. Diarrhea
    c. Vomiting
    d. Flatulence

Answer: a

16. **The most appropriate goal of the nursing diagnosis of pain related to surgery and illness is that the child will**
    a. Require no pain medication
    b. Express less anxiety
    c. Report reduced pain
    d. Understand the pain process

Answer: c

17. **The nurse recognizes that the pain a child experiences will increase with**
    a. The presence of the child's parents
    b. Anxiety
    c. Sleep
    d. Constipation

Answer: b

18. **When administering analgesics to a child, the appropriate analgesic antagonist to have on hand is**
    a. Naproxen
    b. Nubain
    c. Naloxone
    d. Numorphan

Answer: c

19. **Clinical signs which indicate the development of respiratory depression in children receiving opioid analgesics include**
    a. Hyperexcitability and hyperventilation
    b. Sleepiness, small pupils, and shallow breathing
    c. Intractable nausea and vomiting
    d. Sedation, nausea, vomiting, and constipation

Answer: b

20. **When a child has been taking narcotics for severe pain over a period of several days, an increased amount of the narcotic may need to be used because the child develops**
    a. Sensitivity to the narcotic
    b. Intolerance to the narcotic
    c. Tolerance to the narcotic
    d. Insensitivity to the narcotic

Answer: c

21. **The single most powerful nonpharmacologic method of pain relief available for children is**
    a. The parents' presence
    b. Hypnosis
    c. Cutaneous stimulation
    d. Application of heat and cold

Answer: a

22. **When working with an infant who is expressing pain and discomfort, an effective nonpharmacologic method of pain relief that the nurse can employ is**
    a. Playing classical music
    b. Use of a colorful mobile
    c. Use of a pacifier
    d. Electroanalgesia

Answer: c

23. **A process used by the nurse with an 8-year-old child, in which the child is encouraged to focus in on a favorite place, event, or story to reduce pain, is**
    a. Abdominal breathing
    b. Imagery
    c. Hypnosis
    d. Relaxation

Answer: b

24. **When a child is being prepared for a painful procedure such as burn debridement, the physician will most likely order the administration of**
    a. NSAIDs
    b. NSAIDs and an opioid analgesic
    c. Analgesia and anxiolysis
    d. A narcotic analgesic and naloxone

Answer: c

25. **Thirty minutes after administering an opioid analgesic, the nurse notes a decrease in B/P from 124/80 to 104/72, a decrease in respirations from 45 to 30, and a decrease in pulse from 140 to 90. The nurse recognizes the analgesic was**
    a. Effective at relieving pain
    b. Not strong enough to relieve the pain
    c. Too large of a dosage for this child
    d. A threat to the child's respiratory status

Answer: a

8

ALTERATIONS IN FLUID, ELECTROLYTE, AND ACID–BASE BALANCE

1. **In a child who has extracellular volume excess, important nursing assessment activities include**
   a. Daily weights and measurement of intake and output
   b. Checking for orthostatic hypotension
   c. Taking temperature and blood pressure every 3 to 4 hours
   d. Determination of the aldosterone level

   Answer: a

2. **When a child has rapid weight gain, fluid intake greater than fluid output, and a bounding pulse, the nursing diagnosis is**
   a. Fluid volume deficit
   b. Fluid volume excess
   c. Altered cardiac output
   d. Potential for dehydration

   Answer: b

3. **An essential assessment in a child who has extracellular fluid volume deficit is**
   a. Pupillary response
   b. Pedal pulses
   c. Daily weights
   d. Gag reflex

   Answer: c

4. **If a child has rapid weight loss, postural hypotension, delayed capillary filling time, and decreased skin turgor, the nursing diagnosis is**
   a. Fluid volume excess
   b. Altered nutrition, less than body requires
   c. High risk for altered skin integrity
   d. Fluid volume deficit

   Answer: d

5. **To determine if a child is hypernatremic, the nurse should**
   a. Monitor serum sodium level measure intake and output, and urine specific gravity
   b. Restrict fluid intake for 12 hours, and then monitor serum sodium level
   c. Monitor blood pressure, pulse, and respirations every 15 minutes
   d. Do a complete neuro check every 30 minutes

   Answer: a

6. **To monitor a hypernatremic child's response to therapy, the nurse should**
   a. Determine the serum sodium level and the urine specific gravity
   b. Restrict fluid intake for 12 hours, and then determine the serum sodium level
   c. Assess blood pressure, pulse, and respirations every 15 minutes
   d. Frequently assess level of consciousness

   Answer: d

7. An appropriate nursing diagnosis for the hypernatremic child is
   a. High risk for injury related to edema
   b. High risk for injury related to level of consciousness
   c. High risk for altered skin integrity related to edema
   d. High risk for altered skin integrity related to lethargy

Answer: b

8. As most children develop dehydration from gastroenteritis, repeated vomiting, and diarrhea, the nurse realizes that clinical dehydration is a combination of
   a. Body fluid volume that is too high and body fluids that are too concentrated
   b. Extracellular fluid volume excess and altered level of consciousness
   c. Extracellular fluid volume deficit and hypernatremia
   d. Body fluid volume that is too low and hypernatremia

Answer: c

9. In teaching parents effective oral rehydration of their child who has diarrhea and is mildly dehydrated, the nurse stresses diluting fluids such as apple juice and cola to half-strength because
   a. Too highly concentrated solutions can increase the severity of diarrhea
   b. Too much sugar can increase the severity of diarrhea
   c. Mildly dehydrated children need more fluid than moderately dehydrated children
   d. The full-strength mixture will cause gas

Answer: a

10. A frantic mother has just brought her lethargic infant into the emergency room. The baby has had diarrhea for the past 2 days and has not been offered any fluids other than water to drink. Your potential nursing diagnosis is
    a. High risk for injury related to hypotension
    b. Self-care deficit related to lethargy
    c. Knowledge deficit (parent) regarding home management of diarrhea
    d. Fluid volume excess

Answer: c

11. A child has developed hyponatremia as a result of being given tap water to replace fluids lost through diarrhea. The nurse should
    a. Advise the parents to always bring the child to the hospital whenever diarrhea is present
    b. Investigate for further signs of child abuse
    c. Report the parents to social rehabilitation services
    d. Teach the parents to replace body fluids with oral electrolyte solutions

Answer: d

12. In giving a report to the nursing assistant who will be bathing a child with edema, the nurse cautions that the edematous skin is very fragile because edema
    a. Pushes the cells farther apart than normal
    b. Is caused by hydrostatic pressure
    c. Causes swelling of the muscle
    d. Makes the skin thin and shiny

Answer: a

13. Essential daily assessments of a child with edema caused by extracellular fluid volume excess include
    a. Serial blood pressure readings
    b. Determination of electrolyte levels
    c. Weight and intake and output
    d. Determination of the aldosterone level

Answer: c

14. An important nursing diagnosis for the child who is hypocalcemic is
    a. High risk for increased cardiac output related to arrhythmias
    b. High risk for injury related to neuromuscular excitability
    c. Anxiety related to knowledge deficit
    d. Muscle cramps related to hypocalcemia

Answer: b

15. In children with hypercalcemia, vitamin D supplementation should be avoided because

a. It increases urinary output
b. The urine must be kept acidic
c. Vitamin D causes kidney stones which can block ureters
d. It increases the absorption of calcium from the intestinal tract

Answer: d

16. **In the maintenance of acid-base balance, the kidneys excrete metabolic acids and the lungs excrete**
    a. Carbonic acids
    b. Nonbicarbonate buffers
    c. Carbon dioxide
    d. Phosphate ions

Answer: a

17. **Decreased blood pH levels below the normal range for children of 7.37 to 7.43 are associated with a condition called**
    a. Acidemia
    b. Alkalemia
    c. Buffer imbalance
    d. Base imbalance

Answer: a

18. **Following surgery, a child's breathing is slow and shallow. The nurse encourages return to a normal breathing pattern to prevent**
    a. Carbonic acid from accumulating in the blood
    b. A decrease in P_{CO_2}
    c. An increase in bicarbonate
    d. The pH of the blood from becoming alkalemic

Answer: a

19. **When a child begins to hyperventilate, the nurse attempts to slow the breathing down to normal to prevent**
    a. Metabolic alkalosis
    b. Metabolic acidosis
    c. Respiratory alkalosis
    d. Respiratory acidosis

Answer: c

20. **The child who is being treated for salicylate poisoning is at high risk for developing**
    a. Respiratory alkalosis
    b. Respiratory acidosis

c. Metabolic alkalosis
d. Metabolic acidosis

Answer: a

21. **When the body tries to compensate for metabolic acidosis, the respirations take on a characteristic pattern described as**
    a. Apnea
    b. Kussmaul's respiration
    c. Hyperventilation
    d. Cheyne-Stokes respiration

Answer: b

22. **In a child who does not produce adequate amounts of urine (oliguria), the potential is great for the development of**
    a. Metabolic acidosis
    b. Metabolic alkalosis
    c. Respiratory acidosis
    d. Respiratory alkalosis

Answer: a

23. **The chemoreceptors in the brain and arteries are stimulated and respiratory compensation of metabolic acidosis occurs when the**
    a. H_{CO_3} increases above normal levels
    b. P_{CO_2} increases above normal levels
    c. pH of the blood increases above normal
    d. pH of the blood decreases below normal

Answer: d

24. **In assessing laboratory values of the child with metabolic alkalosis, the nurse notes increased H_{CO_3}, pH, and normal P_{CO_2}, indicating**
    a. Acute uncompensated metabolic alkalosis
    b. Partially compensated metabolic alkalosis
    c. Fully compensated metabolic alkalosis
    d. A shift toward metabolic acidosis

Answer: a

25. **In the child with metabolic alkalosis, the body compensates for this condition by**
    a. Vomiting and diarrhea
    b. Retention of bicarbonate
    c. Retention of carbonic acid
    d. Increased renal absorption of bicarbonate

Answer: c

9

ALTERATIONS IN IMMUNE FUNCTION

1. **Aquired immunity is not fully developed until a child is approximately**
   a. 2 years of age
   b. 4 years of age
   c. 6 years of age
   d. 8 years of age
   Answer: c

2. **How long after a child has been exposed to an invasion of foreign substances or antigens does it take for the primary immune response to occur?**
   a. 1 day
   b. 3 days
   c. 5 days
   d. 7 days
   Answer: b

3. **Children under the age of 6 are more susceptible to illness than older children because**
   a. The inflammatory and phagocytic properties of immunity are absent
   b. Their immune systems cannot identify antigens
   c. Their T-lymphocytes develop very slowly
   d. They have a limited supply of immunoglobulins
   Answer: d

4. **Symptoms of B-cell disorders usually become apparent after**
   a. 3 days
   b. 1 month
   c. 3 months
   d. 6 months
   Answer: c

5. **A significant clinical finding in a 3-month-old infant with severe combined immunodeficiency disease is**
   a. Sudden weight gain
   b. Bleeding tendency
   c. Eczema
   d. Resistant oral candidiasis
   Answer: d

6. **In caring for a child with SCID, the nurse performs a thorough physical assessment and determines the following to be significant findings:**
   a. Weight and height above the average for age
   b. Hepatomegaly and lymphadenopathy
   c. Pink mucous membranes
   d. Increased anterior-posterior diameter of the chest
   Answer: b

7. **What is the appropriate nursing diagnosis for an infant admitted with severe combined immuno-deficiency disease (SCID)?**
   a. Risk for alteration of body temperature
   b. Risk for fluid volume deficit
   c. Risk for infection
   d. Altered bowel elimination
   Answer: c

8. **In teaching parents of a child with SCID about potential side effects of long-term use of antibiotics, the nurse explains the need to monitor for**
   a. Thrush infections in the mouth
   b. An increase in temperature
   c. Toughening of the skin
   d. Weight gain
   Answer: a

9. **In teaching parents of a child with Wiskott-Aldrich syndrome to understand the transmission of the disease, the nurse emphasizes**
   a. The prognosis of the disease is good with aggressive antibiotic therapy
   b. The disease is passed on from parent to child
   c. The cause of the disease is unknown
   d. Corticosteroid therapy may put the disease in remission
   Answer: b

10. **The leading cause of immune disease in infants and children, and the leading cause of death in children between 1 and 4, is**
    a. Leukemia
    b. SCID
    c. Cancer
    d. HIV infection
    Answer: d

11. **Most newly reported cases of HIV in children are a result of**
    a. Blood transfusions
    b. Perinatal transmission
    c. Transplant of an organ
    d. Unknown causes
    Answer: b

12. **A child born to an HIV-positive mother is considered free of HIV after**
    a. Two negative PCR tests
    b. Two consecutive negative ELISA tests
    c. One negative ELISA test
    d. One negative PCR test
    Answer: b

13. **The risk for perinatal transmission of HIV is significantly reduced if the infected mother receives**
    a. Fetal blood transfusions during pregnancy
    b. Gamma globulin during pregnancy
    c. Zidovudine (ZDV) during pregnancy
    d. Blood transfusions during pregnancy
    Answer: c

14. **A grandmother who has custody of a 21-month-old granddaughter with AIDS is visiting and asks the nurse, "What is the white stuff all over her mouth?" How should the nurse respond?**
    a. "It's just curdled milk from her last bottle."
    b. "That's some medication I just gave her."
    c. "They're Koplik spots inside her cheeks and on her tongue."
    d. "She's developed a thrush infection."
    Answer: d

15. **In the discharge teaching to be done with the family of a school-age child with AIDS, what information needs to be provided to parents?**
    a. School can be resumed without restrictions as long as the physician approves
    b. School will be limited to part-time attendance only
    c. The child will have to be home-schooled
    d. A nurse must accompany the child to school
    Answer: a

16. **What is the most critical component of the discharge teaching that needs to be done with the family of a child with AIDS?**
    a. Providing them with a list of available community resources
    b. Explaining the signs and symptoms of an infection

c. Discussing methods of maintaining the child's nutritional intake

d. Reviewing methods of transmission

Answer: b

17. **What disorder results in the characteristic butterfly rash on the face of an adolescent?**

a. DiGeorge syndrome

b. Wiskott-Aldrich syndrome

c. AIDS

d. Systemic lupus erythematosus

Answer: d

18. **In teaching an adolescent girl about managing her systemic lupus erythematosus, the nurse emphasizes**

a. To use a heavy makeup base when going out in the sun

b. A daily physical activity program

c. The need to increase fluid intake

d. Avoiding sunlight and using sun protection

Answer: d

19. **The inflammation, pain, and swelling of the joints of a child with juvenile rheumatoid arthritis (JRA) can result in**

a. Atrophy of the joints and surrounding muscle

b. Leakage of fluid from the synovial cavity into the tissue

c. Buildup of scar tissue which limits range of motion

d. Systemic rash and itching

Answer: c

20. **Children with JRA who do not respond to aspirin or nonsteroidal anti-inflammatory drugs may be treated with**

a. Corticosteroids

b. Immune globulin

c. Sulfasalazine and methotrexate

d. Antibiotics

Answer: c

21. **In reviewing the essentials of a well-balanced diet with parents of a child with JRA, the nurse emphasizes**

a. The need to balance caloric intake with activity to prevent weight gain

b. Increasing the number of fruit and vegetable servings every day

c. Decreasing meat intake once activity decreases

d. Increasing milk and milk product intake

Answer: a

22. **The nurse teaches the parents and child who has had a severe or systemic reaction to a bee or wasp sting the need to**

a. Avoid bees and wasps

b. Avoid contact with all insects

c. Use massive amounts of insect repellant before going outside

d. Have a fresh adrenaline kit on hand at all times

Answer: d

23. **Children who are at highest risk for developing latex allergies are those with**

a. Dermatitis

b. Type A blood

c. Asthma

d. Congenital urinary tract anomalies

Answer: d

24. **In teaching parents about safe latex-free toys for children, the nurse suggests**

a. That all toys be taken away from the child

b. Only cloth, vinyl, and plastic toys be used

c. All rubber toys be cleaned with alcohol before the child handles them

d. The child be limited to only 30 minutes or less of playtime with toys

Answer: b

25. **The parents of a child with latex allergies are told to caution all visitors to avoid giving the child**

a. Chewing gum

b. Fresh fruits

c. Stuffed animals

d. Ice cream

Answer: a

10

INFECTIOUS AND
COMMUNICABLE DISEASES

1. **A vaccine that contains an inactive microorganism still capable of inducing the human body to produce antibodies is called a**
   a. Killed virus vaccine
   b. Live virus vaccine
   c. Toxoid
   d. Conjugated vaccine

   Answer: a

2. **A vaccine that contains a microorganism in a weakened form is called a**
   a. Killed virus vaccine
   b. Recombinant form vaccine
   c. Toxoid
   d. Conjugated vaccine

   Answer: b

3. **A vaccine that contains a microorganism that has been genetically altered is called a(n)**
   a. Killed virus vaccine
   b. Inactivated vaccine
   c. Recombinant form vaccine
   d. Conjugated vaccine

   Answer: c

4. **A vaccine which contains a microorganism that is joined with another substance to increase immune response is called a(n)**
   a. Killed virus vaccine
   b. Inactivated vaccine
   c. Toxoid
   d. Conjugated vaccine

   Answer: d

5. **An example of a live virus vaccine is the**
   a. Tetanus toxoid
   b. Hepatitis B vaccine
   c. Varicella vaccine
   d. Inactivated poliovirus vaccine

   Answer: a

6. **An example of a killed virus vaccine is the**
   a. Tetanus toxoid
   b. Hepatitis B vaccine
   c. *Haemophilus influenza* type B vaccine
   d. Inactivated poliovirus vaccine

   Answer: d

7. **An example of a vaccine in the conjugated form is the**
   a. Tetanus toxoid
   b. Hepatitis B vaccine
   c. *Haemophilus influenza* type B vaccine
   d. Inactivated poliovirus vaccine

   Answer: c

8. **When antibodies are produced in an animal or human host and then given to a child, the child acquires**
   a. Active immunity
   b. Passive immunity
   c. A secondary infection
   d. A primary infection

   Answer: b

9. **According to the American Academy of Pediatrics and the American Academy of Family Practitioners, the Hepatitis B series should ideally be**
   a. Initiated at birth and completed by 6 months
   b. Initiated at birth and completed by 6 years
   c. Initiated at 6 months and completed by 1 year
   d. Initiated at 1 year and completed by 18 months

   Answer: a

10. **According to the American Academy of Pediatrics and the American Academy of Family Practitioners, the measles, mumps, and rubella series should ideally be**
    a. Initiated at birth and completed by 6 months
    b. Initiated at 12 months and completed by 6 years
    c. Initiated at 6 months and completed by 1 year
    d. Initiated at 1 year and completed by 18 months

    Answer: b

11. **The influenza vaccine is currently recommended for**
    a. All children between the ages of 2 and 16
    b. Children with chronic pulmonary or cardiac disease
    c. Children with renal impairment
    d. Only those children with a history of frequent influenza

    Answer: b

12. **When children have missed several vaccines, the nurse in the immunization clinic should**
    a. Initiate the first of the missed vaccines and set up several catch-up appointments
    b. Give as many compatible vaccines at once to complete the immunization schedule
    c. Contact the child's primary physician for orders
    d. Administer a series of immune globulin injections and half of the missing vaccines

    Answer: b

13. **The poliovirus vaccine is contraindicated for persons with an allergy to**
    a. Neomycin
    b. Penicillin
    c. Aspirin
    d. Eggs

    Answer: a

14. **In teaching parents about side effects of the MMR vaccine, the nurse explains that the child may develop an elevated temperature**
    a. Within the first 24 hours
    b. Approximately 48 hours following the vaccine
    c. 3 to 5 days following the vaccine
    d. 5 to 12 days following the vaccine

    Answer: d

15. **The nurse gives explicit directions to parents and caregivers to wash hands carefully after every diaper change for the first month after this particular vaccine:**
    a. Inactivated poliovirus
    b. Oral poliovirus
    c. Varicella
    d. Tetanus toxoid

    Answer: b

16. **The appropriate emergency medication for vaccine anaphylaxis is**
    a. Epinephrine 1:100
    b. Epinephrine 1:1000
    c. Morphine sulfate
    d. Phenobarbital

    Answer: b

17. **Which one of the following communicable diseases must be reported to the CDC?**
    a. Varicella
    b. Diphtheria
    c. Fifth disease
    d. Lyme disease

    Answer: b

18. **A potential complication of diphtheria which must be monitored for is**
    a. Liver disease
    b. Memory loss
    c. Airway obstruction
    d. Hypothermia

    Answer: c

19. **The nurse assesses a child with flu-like symptoms, circumoral pallor, and a ruddy facial rash. These symptoms are most indicative of**
    a. Fifth disease
    b. Varicella
    c. Mumps
    d. Hepatitis B

    Answer: a

20. **Hepatitis B is transmitted primarily through**
    a. Contaminated fluid
    b. Body fluids
    c. Airborne route
    d. Skin contact

    Answer: b

21. **The passage of an infectious disease through contaminated utensils is an example of what type of transmission?**
    a. Active
    b. Inactive
    c. Direct
    d. Indirect

    Answer: d

22. **The passage of an infectious disease through physical contact between two persons is an example of what type of transmission?**
    a. Active
    b. Inactive
    c. Direct
    d. Indirect

    Answer: c

23. **Passive immunity that is transferred from mother to infant is referred to as**
    a. Paternal immunity
    b. Fetal immunity
    c. Maternal immunity
    d. Transplacental immunity

    Answer: d

24. **An infection which a person may acquire while in a hospital is called a(n)**
    a. Institutional infection
    b. Nosocomial infection
    c. Passive infection
    d. Transferred infection

    Answer: b

25. **The most common routes for transfer of infection in young children are**
    a. Fecal-oral and respiratory routes
    b. Skin and fecal routes
    c. Urinary tract and gastrointestinal routes
    d. Nasal and ear routes

    Answer: a

11

ALTERATIONS IN
RESPIRATORY FUNCTION

1. **There is a greater potential for an airway obstruction in a small child than an adult because**
   a. A child cannot breathe through the mouth
   b. A child has fewer functional muscles in the airway
   c. The epiglottis in a child is shorter than in an adult
   d. The larynx and glottis are much lower in the neck than in an adult

   Answer: b

2. **In addition to signs of respiratory distress, the initial clinical manifestations of respiratory failure include**
   a. Tachycardia and tachypnea
   b. Bradycardia and bradypnea
   c. Cyanosis and dyspnea
   d. Hot and flushed skin

   Answer: a

3. **In preparing parents of an infant with apnea for discharge, it is essential that the parents learn**
   a. Transcutaneous P_{O_2} and P_{CO_2}
   b. How to feed the infant to prevent apneic episodes
   c. Cardiopulmonary resuscitation
   d. Where to buy an oscillating water bed

   Answer: c

4. **In assisting parents to deal with their infant's death from SIDS, the nurse encourages them to attend**
   a. Parenting classes
   b. Screenings for their remaining children
   c. Legal advisory sessions
   d. The SIDS Alliance

   Answer: d

5. **Arterial blood gas levels indicative of respiratory failure are**
   a. P_{O_2} and P_{CO_2} greater than 50 mm Hg
   b. P_{CO_2} greater than a 50 mm Hg and pH greater than 7.5
   c. P_{O_2} greater than 50 mm Hg and pH less than 7.5
   d. P_{O_2} less than 50 mm Hg and P_{CO_2} greater than 50 mm Hg

   Anwer: d

6. **In caring for a child with respiratory failure, the nurse monitors for imminent signs of respiratory arrest, which include**
   a. Cyanosis
   b. Nasal flaring
   c. Tachycardia
   d. Retractions

   Answer: a

7. **In caring for the child with respiratory compromise, if the slightest degree of respiratory distress is noted, the nurse**
   a. Inserts an endotracheal tube
   b. Performs an emergency tracheostomy
   c. Immediately elevates the head of the bed
   d. Takes a pulse oximetry reading

   Answer: c

8. **The initial symptoms of laryngotracheobronchitis (croup) include**
   a. Fever and discomfort
   b. Stridor and hoarseness
   c. Drooling and chapped lips
   d. Nausea and vomiting

   Answer: b

9. **A characteristic clinical manifestation of a supraglottic obstruction is**
   a. A sudden decrease in coughing
   b. Acute onset of drooling
   c. A positive throat culture
   d. Bradycardia

   Answer: b

10. **When a child is being treated with corticosteroids for LTB, the nurse must monitor for the following cardiovascular symptom:**
    a. Hypertension
    b. Hypotension
    c. Tachycardia
    d. Bradycardia

    Answer: a

11. **With repeated episodes of bronchospasm, mucosal edema, and mucous plugging, the airway becomes chronically irritated and scarred, resulting in**
    a. A change of voice
    b. Air trapping
    c. A constant tickle in the throat
    d. Postnasal drip

    Answer: b

12. **When assessing a child who has dysphonia, dysphagia, drooling, and distressed respirations, visual inspection of the mouth and throat is**

    a. Done with great care
    b. Imperative
    c. Contraindicated
    d. Hazardous

    Answer: c

13. **When assessing the respiratory status of a child brought in with acute exacerbation of asthma, the nurse notes wheezing during inspiration and expiration phases. This finding is documented as**
    a. Asymptomatic
    b. Mild symptoms
    c. Moderate symptoms
    d. Severe symptoms

    Answer: c

14. **To facilitate breathing and ease respiratory effort, the nurse places the child with asthma symptoms in the following position**
    a. Low-Fowler's
    b. Prone
    c. Semi-Fowler's
    d. Side-lying

    Answer: c

15. **In explaining the importance of maintaining an adequate fluid intake, the nurse discusses the role of hydration in**
    a. Keeping the respiratory secretions alkaline
    b. Increasing the production of mucus in the respiratory tract
    c. Providing extra calories to increase weight
    d. Breaking up trapped mucous plugs in the narrowed airways

    Answer: d

16. **The parents of an asthmatic child realize that various triggers can initiate an asthmatic attack. However, they do not understand what causes the respiratory difficulties. You explain how**
    a. Airflow is obstructed through constriction and narrowing of the airway
    b. Normal protective mechanisms are decreased in response to a stimulus
    c. Anxiety can cause respiratory problems
    d. Psychological problems cause reactive airway responses

    Answer: a

17. **Neonatal respiratory distress syndrome (RDS) results from inadequate**
    a. Hydration of the neonate
    b. Pulmonary surfactant
    c. Oxygenation of the mother during labor
    d. Amounts of amniotic fluid

    Answer: b

18. **In teaching parents why bronchodilators are considered the drug of choice for acute or daily therapy of asthma, the nurse explains that the inhaled drug**
    a. Increases airway inflammation and hyperresponsiveness
    b. Stops wheezing
    c. Relaxes smooth muscle in the airway, which then dilates rapidly
    d. Reduces mucosal edema in the airway, thereby increasing the diameter

    Answer: c

19. **After a 7-year-old child has been placed on theophylline for repeated exacerbations of asthma, the nurse instructs parents to keep the appointments for the serum level checks to ensure that**
    a. The child is not bothered by side effects
    b. The dose is properly adjusted for the child
    c. Glucose metabolism is adequate
    d. Liver enzymes are within normal limits

    Answer: b

20. **The nurse evaluates the effectiveness of positioning and oxygen administration used during an acute asthma exacerbation by**
    a. Assessing dryness and thickness of mucus
    b. Promoting and easing respiratory effort
    c. Monitoring transcutaneous oxygen with the pulse oximeter
    d. Observing for adequate hydration

    Answer: c

21. **In teaching the parents of a child with asthma about the importance of avoiding iced beverages for their child, the nurse explains that**
    a. Iced beverages may precipitate bronchospasm
    b. Iced beverages thicken mucus
    c. Urine specific gravity may be increased
    d. Pulmonary blood vessels may be compromised

    Answer: a

22. **During the treatment of infant respiratory distress syndrome, the parents of the child should be told that the oxygen and positive pressure ventilation may result in**
    a. Hyaline membrane disease
    b. The need for a tracheostomy
    c. Neurological complications
    d. Bronchopulmonary dysplasia

    Answer: d

23. **In teaching the parents of an 18-month-old male who has bronchopulmonary dysplasia the importance of giving the child the prescribed diuretic, the nurse explains that the medication will**
    a. Prevent ascites
    b. Provide specific prophylactic therapy
    c. Enhance urinary elimination
    d. Help remove excess fluid from the lungs

    Answer: d

24. **When caring for an infant with pneumonia, the nurse can ease the pain of coughing by having the child**
    a. Hug a teddy bear, doll, or small pillow
    b. Move to a side-lying position
    c. Take acetaminophen every 4 hours
    d. Sip juice or milk after every coughing episode

    Answer: a

25. **One of the characteristc signs of cystic fibrosis is the presence of**
    a. Hemoptysis
    b. Anorexia
    c. Steatorrhea
    d. Recurrent urinary tract infections

    Answer: c

12

ALTERATIONS IN CARDIOVASCULAR FUNCTION

1. **The closure of the foramen ovale is stimulated during the transition from fetal to pulmonary circulation as a result of**
   a. The birthing process
   b. The newborn's first breath
   c. Increased pressure in the left heart
   d. Closure of the ductus arteriosus

   Answer: c

2. **During stress, fever, or respiratory distress, infants and young children develop tachycardia. This symptom is indicative of**
   a. Congestive heart failure
   b. Weak heart muscles
   c. The heart trying to provide adequate oxyen transport
   d. The heart trying to conserve oxygen consumption

   Answer: c

3. **The nurse caring for the young child in respiratory failure monitors the child for signs of hypoxemia and bradycardia, which can result in**
   a. System overload
   b. Cardiac arrest
   c. Increased cardiac output
   d. Polycythemia

   Answer: b

4. **The child with congestive heart failure must be monitored closely for signs of impending cardiogenic shock, which include**
   a. Weak peripheral pulses and hypotension
   b. Bounding peripheral pulses and hypertension
   c. Nasal flaring and grunting
   d. Retractions with cough

   Answer: a

5. **An infant is to receive digoxin 0.020 mg Q12H. The bottle on hand is labeled "0.05 mg per cc." What is the correct dose to be administered?**
   a. 0.4 cc
   b. 0.8 cc
   c. 1.2 cc
   d. 1.6 cc

   Answer: a

6. **The child who is on diuretic therapy is at greatest risk for which of the following electrolyte imbalances?**
   a. Hypercalcemia
   b. Hypocalcemia
   c. Hyperkalemia
   d. Hypokalemia

   Answer: d

7. **Before giving digoxin to an 18-month-old, the nurse takes the apical pulse for 1 full minute and holds the drug if the pulse is under**
   a. 100
   b. 110
   c. 120
   d. 140

   Answer: a

8. **The parents of a toddler with cyanotic congenital heart disease are asked to bring the child in for a Denver II assessment every 2 to 3 months to evaluate**
   a. Disease management and developmental growth
   b. Respiratory and cardiac function
   c. Nutrition and hydration status
   d. Response to pharmacologic treatment

   Answer: a

9. **The nurse teaches the mother of an infant with congestive heart failure ways to decrease metabolic demands upon the heart during feeding, such as**
   a. Feeding larger volumes less often to conserve energy
   b. Burping the infant less often to reduce stress on the heart
   c. Positioning the infant at a 30 degree angle
   d. Positioning the infant at a 45 degree angle

   Answer: d

10. **In helping parents understand signs of deteriorating cardiac status in their infant with congestive heart failure, the nurse instructs the parents to report**
    a. Increased demand for more frequent feedings by the infant
    b. Increased perspiration and dyspnea with feedings
    c. Sleeping through the night without a feeding
    d. Crying and fussing during the feedings

    Answer: b

11. **A disposable diaper weighing 30 g is placed on an infant and, after voiding, its weight is 52 g. How much urine has the infant voided?**
    a. 11 cc
    b. 22 cc
    c. 41 cc
    d. 82 cc

    Answer: b

12. **An appropriate goal for the nursing diagnosis of activity intolerance related to poor cardiac output is that the infant or child will**
    a. Increase activity tolerance
    b. Experience absence of fatigue during ADLs
    c. Perform all ADLs without undue fatigue
    d. Meet all developmental milestones

    Answer: c

13. **Signs and symptoms which the nurse may assess in the older child diagnosed with congenital heart disease include**
    a. Syncope and arrhythmias
    b. Muscle atrophy and spasms
    c. Tachycardia and hypertension
    d. Facial flushing and edema

    Answer: a

14. **The nurse discusses the valvuloplasty procedure with the parents of a child with a congenital heart defect, explaining the purpose of**
    a. Reattaching of the great arteries with the correct ventricles
    b. Closing of the septal defect by an umbrella device
    c. Repairing of the valve to relieve stenosis by balloon dilation
    d. Placing a constricting band around the pulmonary artery

    Answer: c

15. **What is the medication given intravenously to stimulate closure of the ductus arteriosus in premature infants?**
    a. Prostaglandin E_1
    b. Furosemide
    c. Prednisone
    d. Indomethacin

    Answer: d

16. Following a repair of a cardiac defect, the child is placed on prophylactic antibiotics for an extended period of time primarily to
    a. Keep the child healthy
    b. Boost immunity to everyday pathogens
    c. Prevent genitourinary tract infections
    d. Prevent infective endocarditis

Answer: d

17. In addition to cyanosis, the child having a cyanotic spell will also display
    a. Bradycardia
    b. Tachycardia
    c. Bradypnea
    d. Flushing

Answer: b

18. In implementing emergency procedures with the infant experiencing a cyanotic spell, the nurse positions the infant in a
    a. Prone position
    b. High Fowler's position
    c. Low Fowler's position
    d. Knee-chest position

Answer: d

19. The diagnostic test which measures oxygen saturation and pressures within heart chambers and also identifies anatomic alterations is called
    a. Ultrasonography
    b. Echocardiography
    c. Cardiac catheterization
    d. Magnetic resonance imaging

Answer: c

20. After a 3-year-old returns to his room following a cardiac catheterization, an important nursing intervention which needs to be implemented is
    a. Monitoring the catheterization site for bleeding
    b. Ambulating him early
    c. Restricting fluids until his blood pressure is stable
    d. Comparing blood pressures in the affected and unaffected extremities

Answer: a

21. The parents of a child who has just had a cardiac catheterization ask if they can walk the child down to the play room when he awakens. The nurse informs the parents that the child will be on bedrest for
    a. 3 hours
    b. 6 hours
    c. 12 hours
    d. 24 hours

Answer: b

22. Following correction of an acyanotic congenital heart lesion, parents of a child should be instructed to obtain prophylactic antibiotics prior to
    a. The flu season
    b. Dental procedures
    c. Exposure to preschool
    d. Immunizations

Answer: b

23. The polycythemia present in infants and children with cyanotic congenital heart disease can be best understood as the body's response to
    a. Cardiomegaly
    b. Anemia
    c. Oxygenation need
    d. Decreased cardiac output

Answer: c

24. A nurse caring for a toddler with a cyanotic congenital heart defect can expect the child to have
    a. Elevated hematocrit
    b. Edema
    c. Crackles
    d. Orthopnea

Answer: a

25. Rheumatic fever is an inflammatory disease that follows an initial infection by some strains of
    a. Group A alpha-hemolytic streptococci
    b. Group B alpha-hemolytic streptococci
    c. Group A beta-hemolytic streptococci
    d. Group B beta-hemolytic streptococci

Answer: c

13

ALTERATIONS IN HEMATOLOGIC FUNCTION

1. When a child becomes anemic secondary to hemorrhage, the bone marrow begins to produce large quantitites of red cells. This condition is called
   a. Polycythemia
   b. Hematopoiesis
   c. Thrombocytopenia
   d. Leukopenia

   Answer: a

2. The hemoglobin and hematocrit levels are at highest levels in an infant at age
   a. 6 months
   b. 4 months
   c. 2 months
   d. 1 week

   Answer: d

3. The newborn receives a prophylactic injection of vitamin K at birth because
   a. Red blood cell production is enhanced with vitamin K
   b. Vitamin K is the one nutrient not found in breast or bottle formula
   c. Platelet levels are very low and need vitamin K to be activated
   d. Vitamin K promotes growth of white blood cells

   Answer: c

4. The most common type of nutritional deficiency seen in children today is
   a. Vitamin C deficiency
   b. Calcium deficiency
   c. Iron deficiency anemia
   d. Dehydration

   Answer: c

5. If both parents have the sickle cell trait, with each pregnancy the risk of having a child with the disease is
   a. 25 percent
   b. 50 percent
   c. 75 percent
   d. 100 percent

   Answer: a

6. The best roommate a nurse can select for a 6-year-old who is admitted in sickle cell crisis is a
   a. 6-year-old with ruptured appendix
   b. 7-year-old with congenital heart disease
   c. 5-year-old with diarrhea
   d. 6-year-old with osteomyelitis

   Answer: b

7. **In sickle cell anemia, when does the hemoglobin in the red cell acquire a sickle shape?**
   a. When the red cell is immature
   b. When the red cell is hypoxic
   c. When the hemoglobin is high
   d. When polycythemia is present

Answer: b

8. **The painful crises of children with a sickle cell disorder are caused by**
   a. Occlusion of small blood vessels
   b. Thickened blood
   c. Pooling of blood in the spleen
   d. Defective synthesis of hemoglobin

Answer: a

9. **Nursing interventions which need to be considered in developing a care plan for a 7-year-old admitted in vaso-occlusive sickle cell crisis include**
   a. Oxygenation, assessment of infection, and factor VIII replacement
   b. Pain management, administering heparin, and hydration
   c. Hydration, rest, and pain management
   d. Oxygenation, administering antibiotics, and factor IX replacement

Answer: c

10. **A clinic nurse teaching parents whose children have sickle cell disease stresses the need for them to**
    a. Provide foods high in iron
    b. Administer the medications ordered
    c. Encourage participation in physical activities
    d. Give large amounts of fluids

Answer: d

11. **Symptoms of what blood disorder include purpura, petechiae, and thrombocytopenia and pancytopenia?**
    a. Hemophilia
    b. Normocytic anemia
    c. Sickle cell anemia
    d. Aplastic anemia

Answer: d

12. **The nurse preparing a discharge teaching plan for the hemophiliac child and his family emphasizes recognition of the following signs of internal bleeding:**
    a. Loss of appetite without loss of weight
    b. Joint pain and swelling and abdominal pain
    c. Increase in thirst and urination
    d. Loss of muscle mass surrounding joints

Answer: b

13. **With nutritional counseling being an important aspect of managing a child with sickle cell disease, what type of diet does a nurse emphasize to both parents and child?**
    a. High-protein, high-calorie
    b. High-mineral, low-fat
    c. High-protein, low-carbohydrate
    d. High-fiber, high-iron

Answer: a

14. **The nurse encourages the mother of a 6-month-old baby to begin feeding the infant solid foods at this time because**
    a. They help control the weight of the baby
    b. The child is less picky at this age
    c. Neonatal iron stores are depleted by this age
    d. Bone marrow activity is depressed at this age

Answer: c

15. **An 8-month-old baby has been diagnosed with iron deficiency anemia. The nurse teaches the mother of the infant to add what food to the daily diet?**
    a. Mineral-fortified cereal
    b. Orange juice
    c. Whole milk
    d. Strained beef

Answer: a

16. **When instructing parents on the use of iron supplements for children with iron deficiency anemia, the nurse cautions that the supplements**
    a. Should be given with milk
    b. Need to be diluted before administration
    c. Will turn the child's stools black
    d. Tend to discolor the buccal mucosa

Answer: c

17. **A blood disorder which is predominant among children of Mediterranean origin is**
    a. Aplastic anemia
    b. Sickle cell anemia
    c. ß-thalassemia
    d. Von Willebrand's disease

    Answer: c

18. **When bone marrow is taken from a child before undergoing chemotherapy, and reinfused after the treatment, the bone marrow transplantation is referred to as**
    a. Transfusion therapy
    b. Allogenic
    c. Isogenic
    d. Autologous

    Answer: d

19. **When a child with Cooley's anemia develops hemosiderosis as a result of frequent transfusions, the body stores**
    a. Calcium in the joints
    b. Glycogen in the liver
    c. Magnesium in the fat tissue
    d. Iron in tissues and organs

    Answer: d

20. **In caring for the child with Cooley's anemia, the nurse recognizes the need to treat hemosiderosis with**
    a. Deferoxamine and vitamin C
    b. Prolonged bedrest
    c. Alternating cold and hot packs
    d. Foods rich in iron

    Answer: a

21. **To ensure that the child with hemophilia meets the appropriate developmental landmarks, the nurse encourages parents to involve the child in**
    a. Competitive sports with other children in the same age group
    b. Low-impact sports such as swimming and hiking
    c. Sedentary activities such as reading and watching TV
    d. Contact sports to increase feelings of normalcy

    Answer: b

22. **Adolescent girls with Von Willebrand's disease may have increased menstrual bleeding, which is referred to as**
    a. Erythropoiesis
    b. Amenorrhea
    c. Menorrhagia
    d. Hematopoiesis

    Answer: c

23. **When the child with hemophilia is bleeding into tissues of the neck, mouth, or chest, the child is at high risk for**
    a. Loss of consciousness
    b. Impending shock
    c. Infection
    d. Airway obstruction

    Answer: d

24. **The most appropriate nursing diagnosis that can be selected for a 3-year-old with hemophilia who is experiencing hemarthrosis is**
    a. Knowledge deficit related to disease management
    b. High risk for impaired skin integrity related to cast wear
    c. Alteration in mobility, potential joint contractures
    d. Alteration in nutrition, more than body requirements

    Answer: c

25. **A nursing intervention that needs to be implemented in caring for a child with hemophilia who is bleeding actively into his left knee joint is**
    a. Skin traction
    b. Active range-of-motion exercises
    c. Warm packs
    d. Immobilization

    Answer: d

14

ALTERATIONS IN CELLULAR GROWTH

1. **The primary cause of cancer in children is related to the following:**
   a. Embryonic changes
   b. Exposure to toxins in the environment
   c. Lifestyle
   d. Stress

   Answer: a

2. **The nurse caring for the immunosuppressed child must monitor for the presence of overwhelming infection (septic shock), characterized by**
   a. Hypertension, bradycardia, and bradypnea
   b. Hemorrhage caused by DIC and accompanied by hypotension
   c. Increased intracranial pressure and seizures
   d. Circulatory failure, inadequate tissue perfusion, and hypotension

   Answer: d

3. **The nurse caring for the child with mild to moderate thrombocytopenia teaches the parents to**
   a. Give Septra as ordered
   b. Protect the child's body from bruising
   c. Keep the child well hydrated
   d. Promote good oral hygiene

   Answer: b

4. **When assessing the child who is being treated for cancer, it is important to remember that hair loss, surgical scars, and cushingoid changes are**
   a. Discussed only if the child brings up concerns
   b. The result of the child's immature immune system
   c. Threats to the child's body image
   d. Easier for a child to accept than an adult

   Answer: c

5. **You have assessed a 4-year-old child with body image disturbances. To encourage the child to express feelings about the altered part and to reinforce the positive aspects of change, you**
   a. Confront the child with the change
   b. Avoid talking about the affected area
   c. Discuss ways of compensating for the loss
   d. Use dolls and drawings as therapeutic play

   Answer: d

6. **In working with families of a child newly diagnosed with cancer, the nurse recognizes that when providing information about the disease process and treatment options,**
   a. Always give written materials
   b. Repeat information over time, verbally and in writing
   c. Discuss the effect of anxiety on the retention of knowledge
   d. Respect their need to avoid direct confrontation

   Answer: b

7. It is essential for the nurse to perform a thorough developmental assessment of a child with cancer before treatment and at regular intervals during treatment to evaluate
   a. Progress made during treatment and long-term effects of treatment
   b. The cost-effectiveness of the treatment
   c. The effect of the cancer on the family roles
   d. Environmental changes during treatment

   Answer: a

8. The primary focus on the ongoing physiologic nursing assessment of the child undergoing active treatment for cancer centers on the
   a. Child's knowledge of the cancer and the treatments
   b. Stress and coping patterns of the child and the family
   c. Side effects of the treatment on the child
   d. Ongoing psychosocial needs of the child and the family

   Answer: c

9. The normal parental reaction to having a child with cancer is powerlessness. The nurse can promote a greater sense of parental control by
   a. Helping them to understand why the child keeps relapsing
   b. Including, informing, and supporting them throughout treatment
   c. Referral to the team's psychologist
   d. Having the oncologist discuss treatment, long-term effects, and outcomes

   Answer: b

10. When treating the pain associated with cancer, the expected outcome is that the child experiences pain reduction that allows the child to
    a. Rest and sleep as appropriate for age
    b. Relax and use deep breathing
    c. Feel rested, as expressed by report
    d. Interact appropriately and to gain rest

    Answer: d

11. The nurse working with the child who is nauseated from chemotherapy can ensure optimal nutritional intake by
    a. Administering antiemetic drugs on a regular basis
    b. Allowing the child to eat in a large, well-lit room
    c. Offer general trays with a larger selection of foods to try
    d. Offering favorite foods when nauseated

    Answer: a

12. In order to facilitate adaptive coping mechanisms in the child with cancer, the nurse can
    a. Allow for expression of angry feelings
    b. Ignore the child during angry outbursts
    c. Observe the child for destructive behavior
    d. Help the child to fantasize

    Answer: a

13. You are in the home evaluating the nutritional status of a child who has cancer. One objective measure for determining the maintenance of adequate nutritional intake is
    a. Having the child and/or parents keep a daily dietary log
    b. Taking a thorough nutrition history now and at each follow-up visit
    c. Checking the child's weight for height now and at each follow-up visit
    d. Promoting normal hygiene

    Answer: c

14. The parents of a 7-year-old child who has just finished a course of chemotherapy are concerned about having her return to her normal school/play routine. The nurse promotes adaptation by discussing
    a. The best time to begin extracurricular activities
    b. Ways to save energy for play and school
    c. When to see peers, if too tired to attend school
    d. The possibility of taking naps at school

    Answer: b

15. **You are caring for a 14-month-old child who has a brain tumor. As part of baseline prior to surgery, the nurse should**
    a. Fit the child's head for a surgical cap
    b. Measure the child's head circumference and assess the anterior fontanel
    c. Assess the status of both the anterior and the posterior fontanels
    d. Obtain a culture of the scalp tissue

Answer: b

16. **An essential nursing strategy when working with the child with a neuroblastoma is to assess the child for**
    a. Urine catecholamines
    b. Pressure on major blood vessels
    c. Anemia and thrombocytopenia
    d. Tumor stage

Answer: b

17. **The most appropirate nursing diagnosis for the child who has just had a limb amputated because of bone cancer is**
    a. Disturbed body image
    b. Phantom pain
    c. Impaired wound healing
    d. Impaired limb function

Answer: a

18. **The most common form of leukemia in children is acute**
    a. Nonlymphocytic leukemia
    b. Myelogenous leukemia
    c. Lymphocytic leukemia
    d. Lymphoblastic leukemia

Answer: c

19. **When a child with leukemia is receiving cyclophosphamide, the nurse should pay special attention to**
    a. Hematuria
    b. Renal function
    c. Bone marrow suppression
    d. Neurologic problems

Answer: b

20. **When working with children who have soft tissue tumors, the nurse avoids using palpation to assess the tumor because**
    a. Such manipulation causes pain
    b. The lymph nodes may clog
    c. Only the physician can palpate
    d. The tumor may spread if palpation is done

Answer: d

21. **In providing home care instructions for the parents of a child with cancer, the nurse emphasizes good handwashing technique because**
    a. The cancer cells live outside of the body
    b. The home environment is not as clean as the hospital
    c. Handwashing will increase the parents' feelings of security
    d. Children with cancer are severely immunosuppressed

Answer: d

22. **The nurse performing an assessment on a child with a brain tumor will include assessment of**
    a. Level of consciousness and pupils (shape, size, and response to light)
    b. Cranial nerves
    c. Motor ability and sixth cranial nerve involvement
    d. Urinary output and specific gravity

Answer: a

23. **In discussing the primary purpose of infusing large volumes of intravenous fluids with the chemotherapy medication, the nurse explains to parents that the**
    a. Child will have less nausea when fully hydrated
    b. Fluids help flush the cancerous cell fragments out of the body
    c. Side effects of the drugs are thirst
    d. By diluting the chemotherapeutic drug in the body, it is more effective

Answer: b

24. **While a child is receiving chemotherapy treatments, the nurse instructs parents to observe for and report which of the following significant observations?**
    a. Increase in urinary output
    b. Fatigue
    c. Redness, warmth, and tenderness at the central line site
    d. Excessive thirst

    Answer: c

25. **When administering chemotherapeutic drugs to the child with cancer, the nurse monitors the IV site closely to avoid leakage of the drug into the soft tissue surrounding the site. This potential complication is referred to as**
    a. Metastasis
    b. Thrombocytopenia
    c. Myelosuppression
    d. Extravasation

    Answer: d

15

ALTERATIONS IN GASTROINTESTINAL FUNCTION

1. **The new mother becomes concerned over her 1-month-old infant's frequent regurgitation of formula. The nurse explains the infant**
   a. May have an intestinal motility problem
   b. Has a relaxed cardiac sphincter, which is typical of all infants
   c. Should be holding down all the formula by the age of 2 months
   d. Is rejecting the formula; try another formula

   Answer: b

2. **The production of digestive enzymes in infants increases in production by the age of**
   a. 1 to 2 months
   b. 2 to 4 months
   c. 4 to 6 months
   d. 6 to 8 months

   Answer: c

3. **Special precautions which the nurse uses in feeding an infant with a cleft lip or palate include**
   a. Holding the infant in a sitting position
   b. Inserting an NG tube to use for feeding
   c. Use of a specially designed nipple
   d. Raising the infant's feet above heart level during the feeding

   Answer: a

4. **Following the feeding of the child who has had his cleft palate repaired, the nurse**
   a. Permits the child to choose favorite liquids
   b. Cleanses the child's mouth with hydrogen peroxide
   c. Cleanses the child's mouth with water
   d. Allows the child to hold the drinking cup by himself

   Answer: c

5. **In obtaining a history from parents of a 3-week-old suspected of having a pyloric stenosis, what is the most significant comment they make?**
   a. "He fusses after feedings."
   b. "He's difficult to burp."
   c. "He's always drooling formula."
   d. "He seems to vomit with force."

   Answer: d

6. **An infant with a gastrostomy tube in place is offered a pacifier during feedings because**
   a. It meets his non-nutritive sucking needs
   b. Such action facilitates digestion
   c. It decreases the amount of burping that needs to be done
   d. It eliminates the need to place the infant in a side-lying position

   Answer: a

7. **The abdominal assessment of a 1-month-old suspected of having pyloric stenosis will include the following characteristic finding:**
   a. The absence of bowel sounds
   b. Visible peristaltic waves
   c. A rigid abdomen
   d. Passage of excessive flatus

Answer: b

8. **For an infant with gastroesophageal reflux, which of the following assessments is most significant?**
   a. Hypoactive bowel sounds
   b. Flushed, moist skin
   c. A high-pitched cry
   d. Regurgitation of feedings

Answer: d

9. **When pH probe monitoring is necessary, parents need to be advised that its purpose is to**
   a. Assist in the passage of formula through the esophagus
   b. Identify the number of reflux episodes that are occurring
   c. Determine the time it takes for the stomach to empty its contents
   d. Monitor the pH within the stomach

Answer: b

10. **Following the feeding of an infant with gastroesophageal reflux, the nurse positions the infant**
    a. With feet above the heart level
    b. In the side-lying position
    c. With the upper body elevated
    d. In the prone position

Answer: c

11. **In doing a newborn assessment, the best method of evaluating patency of the rectum is for a nurse to**
    a. Feed the newborn formula
    b. Record passage of meconium
    c. Insert a lubricated thermometer
    d. Observe for abdominal distention

Answer: c

12. **Parents of the toddler with an anorectal malformation will need special instructions from the nurse to assist in**
    a. Toilet training
    b. Discipline
    c. Control of temper tantrums
    d. Maintaining nutrition

Answer: a

13. **In caring for the newborn who has had a diaphragmatic hernia repaired, in the immediate postoperative period, the nurse must position the infant**
    a. On the unaffected side
    b. In a semi-Fowler's position
    c. On the affected side
    d. Flat on his back

Answer: c

14. **Although umbilical hernias may concern some parents, it is important to reassure them that most resolve spontaneously by**
    a. The end of the first year
    b. 2 years of age
    c. 3 years of age
    d. 4 years of age

Answer: b

15. **In performing an assessment of a 13-year-old with appendicitis, the nurse palpates the abdomen**
    a. At the end of the examination
    b. At the beginning of the assessment
    c. In the course of doing a review of all systems
    d. Prior to percussion

Answer: a

16. **During the immediate postoperative period, the nurse positions the child who has just had surgery for a ruptured appendix**
    a. On the left side
    b. In the semi-Fowler's position
    c. Flat in bed
    d. In the knee-chest position

Answer: b

17. Which of the following assessment data would the nurse recognize as indicative of initial signs of feeding intolerance in the infant with necrotizing enterocolitis?
    a. Protuberant abdomen and colic
    b. Diarrhea, fever, and irritability
    c. Flatus, diarrhea, and nausea
    d. Vomiting, irritability, and increased gastric residuals

Answer: d

18. The pain associated with Meckel's diverticulum in children is described similarly to the pain of
    a. Peptic ulcer
    b. Appendicitis
    c. Ulcerative colitis
    d. Crohn's disease

Answer: b

19. In working with an adolescent who has inflammatory bowel disease, the most appropriate nursing diagnosis to develop is
    a. Ineffective individual coping
    b. High risk for infection
    c. Noncompliance
    d. Self-esteem disturbance

Answer: d

20. Once able to eat, the diet of a teenager with inflammatory bowel disease should consist of
    a. High-fiber foods
    b. Small frequent meals
    c. Bland foods only
    d. Three meals a day

Answer: b

21. The nurse has assessed a 3-month-old admitted with dehydration and diarrhea, and notes the anterior fontanel to be
    a. Smooth
    b. Flat
    c. Depressed
    d. Bulging

Answer: c

22. The most significant assessment data that the nurse notes in a toddler who is infected with enterobiasis (pinworms) is
    a. Nausea and vomiting
    b. Diarrhea
    c. Elevated temperature
    d. Perianal itching and restlessness

Answer: d

23. In an infant with biliary atresia, the stools are puttylike in consistency and
    a. Tarry-colored
    b. Yellow in color
    c. Clay-colored
    d. Yellow with green streaks

Answer: c

24. After the initial nausea and anorexia associated with hepatitis have passed, the therapeutic diet which is prescribed for the child with hepatitis is
    a. High-protein, high-carbohydrate
    b. Low-protein, low-fat
    c. High-carbohydrate, low-sodium
    d. Low-carbohydrate, high-fiber

Answer: a

25. The therapeutic diet which is prescribed for the child who is exposed to high lead levels is
    a. High in fiber and low in sodium
    b. Low in fat and high in potassium
    c. High in iron and calcium
    d. Low in carbohydrates and iodine

Answer: c

16

ALTERATIONS IN GENITOURINARY FUNCTION

1. When assessing an infant's intake and output, the nurse recognizes that the infant urinary output per kilogram of body weight per hour is approximately
   a. 0.5 to 1 ml/kg/hr
   b. 2 ml/kg/hr
   c. 4 ml/kg/hr
   d. 8 ml/kg/hr

Answer: b

2. In estimating the bladder capacity of a 6-year-old, the nurse determines it to be
   a. 8 ounces
   b. 10 ounces
   c. 12 ounces
   d. 16 ounces

Answer: a

3. The nurse explains to the father of an infant born with a hypospadias that the urethral opening in his child is
   a. Above the anal opening
   b. Absent
   c. On the dorsal surface of the penis
   d. On the ventral surface of the penis

Answer: d

4. When providing discharge teaching to parents of the child who has just had epispadias or hypospadias repair, the nurse emphasizes keeping the urethral stent patent by
   a. Use of the double diapering technique
   b. Irrigating the stent with normal saline three times a day
   c. Encouraging fluid intake
   d. Restraining the child

Answer: c

5. The most accurate diagnostic test for detecting reflux and visualizing bladder structure and function is called the
   a. Voiding cystourethrogram
   b. Renal ultrasound
   c. Diuretic renogram
   d. Radionucleotide scan

Answer: a

6. One of the contributing factors leading to urinary tract infections common in young children is related to
   a. Excessive intake of carbonated beverages
   b. Insufficient water intake to flush kidneys
   c. Voiding patterns of 4 to 6 times per day
   d. Incomplete emptying of the bladder and urinary stasis

Answer: d

7. The nurse instructs a 12-year-old boy on the proper technique for obtaining a urine specimen, and requests an early morning sample because
   a. The urine is more concentrated
   b. The urine is more dilute
   c. Morning is more convenient for the laboratory to analyze the sample
   d. Dysuria is not present in the day

Answer: a

8. In children under 2 years of age who have a fever of unknown origin, it is important to obtain a urine culture so that
   a. Treatments can be started immediately
   b. The presence of a urinary tract infection can be determined
   c. Antibiotics specific for *E. coli* can be started as soon as possible
   d. The degree of dehydration can be determined

Answer: b

9. The mother of an 18-month-old brings the child to the emergency room with symptoms of fever, poor appetite, and strong-smelling urine. The symptoms are indicative of (a)
   a. Gastrointestinal virus
   b. Dehydration
   c. Urinary tract infection
   d. Epispadias

Answer: c

10. The child with recurrent urinary tract infections is at highest risk for
   a. Fistulas
   b. Kidney damage
   c. Bladder cancer
   d. Dehydration

Answer: b

11. When teaching parents and children preventive strategies for UTI, it is important to stress wiping the perineum
   a. From front to back after voiding
   b. From back to front after voiding
   c. With soft toilet paper
   d. After a bowel movement

Answer: a

12. The nurse teaches preventive strategies for UTI to an adolescent girl who is sexually active. An important point to discuss is
   a. Wiping the perineum from front to back
   b. Voiding after sexual intercourse
   c. Discussing her activity with her parents
   d. The use of a condom or other barrier method

Answer: b

13. When obtaining a family history of the child with nocturnal enuresis, the nurse inquires about bedwetting history of parents because
   a. Parents need to show empathy for their child's condition
   b. It is a learned pattern of behavior
   c. There is a familial tendency with nocturnal enuresis
   d. Parents may be subconsciously encouraging enuresis

Answer: c

14. The nurse assesses the child with minimal change nephrotic syndrome (MCNS) and notes significant findings of fluid retention to include
   a. Hypotension
   b. Increase in urine output
   c. Warm and flushed skin
   d. Periorbital edema

Answer: d

15. The child who has MCNS is at high risk for infection related to increased susceptibility and lowered resistance secondary to
   a. Malnutrition
   b. Corticosteroid therapy
   c. Sodium retention
   d. Albumin loss

Answer: b

16. The nurse determines if fluid imbalances need to be adjusted in the dialysis patient by
   a. Analyzing I & O over the last 24 hours
   b. Weighing the child before and after dialysis
   c. Assessing the mucous membranes before dialysis
   d. Determining urine pH before and after dialysis

Answer: b

17. **For the child in acute renal failure (ARF), nursing diagnoses are related to**
    a. Sepsis or drug toxicity
    b. Altered renal tissue perfusion
    c. The cause of the renal failure and its complications
    d. Fluid volume excess or insufficiency

Answer: c

18. **It is important for the nurse to check drug levels of the medications being received by a child in ARF, because**
    a. Of the decrease in the liver's ability to conjugate drugs
    b. The child is oliguric
    c. Of uremic syndrome
    d. The kidney's ability to excrete drugs is impaired

Answer: d

19. **The primary aim in maintaining fluid balance for the child in ARF is to achieve a**
    a. Decrease in serum sodium concentration and increase in weight
    b. Stable serum sodium concentration and decrease in weight
    c. Increase in urine specific gravity and pH
    d. Increase in serum sodium concentration and decrease in weight

Answer: b

20. **The optimal protein intake for an infant in chronic renal failure is**
    a. 2 to 2.5 g/kg/day
    b. 1.5 to 2 g/kg/day
    c. Determined by electrolyte results
    d. Based on potassium and phosphate results

Answer: a

21. **For the child in chronic renal failure, a nursing diagnosis of altered growth and development is related to**
    a. Activity intolerance secondary to fatigue
    b. Decreased liver function
    c. The effect of dialysis on appetite
    d. Decreased caloric intake and metabolic disturbances

Answer: d

22. **The nurse working with the teenage dialysis population will most likely encounter feelings of resentment for being forced to maintain such strict dietary restrictions and dialysis schedule. These behaviors are indicative of the teens'**
    a. Body image disturbance
    b. Need for peer relationships
    c. Need for independence and sense of self
    d. Noncompliance with dietary restrictions

Answer: c

23. **A 6-year-old boy with APSGN is receiving corticosteroids. His parents ask the nurse why his booster shots must be delayed until this treatment has been discontinued for 3 months, and the nurse explains that**
    a. Corticosteroids suppress immune function
    b. Until the kidneys heal, immunizations may not be effective
    c. They need to wait until he no longer retains fluid
    d. Infection can occur prior to that time

Answer: a

24. **The nurse administers diuretics to the young child with APSGN, explaining to the parents that diuretics cause excretion of excess fluids by**
    a. Improving kidney function
    b. Preventing reabsorption of water and sodium
    c. Causing vasodilation
    d. Osmosis

Answer: b

25. **When counseling adolescents about their STDs, the nurse stresses modification of sexual behavior and**
    a. Abstinence
    b. Using oral contraceptives
    c. To be supportive and understanding
    d. The need to treat all sexual partners

Answer: d

17

ALTERATIONS IN EYE, EAR, NOSE, AND THROAT FUNCTION

1. **Since infectious conjunctivitis is extremely contagious, the nurse informs parents of a school-aged child that the child cannot go back to school until**
   a. The child has been taking the prescribed antibiotics for 24 hours
   b. The itching symptoms are gone
   c. The affected conjunctiva is white
   d. The antibiotic course is complete

   Answer: a

2. **The nurse teaching the parents of a newborn feeding techniques cautions the couple not to feed the infant in the supine position because**
   a. The infant needs to be upright in order to digest the formula
   b. Infantile vertigo will occur
   c. There is a greater probability of the infant developing otitis media
   d. There is a greater potential for developing mouth ulcers

   Answer: c

3. **The nurse assesses a child brought into the emergency room with red and purple, tender, puffy eyelids. These symptoms alert the nurse to the potential for**

   a. Child abuse
   b. Periorbital cellulitis
   c. Hyperopia
   d. Glaucoma

   Answer: b

4. **When nurses are caring for preterm neonates who are receiving oxygen therapy, it is imperative that nursing management include**
   a. Protective eyewear
   b. Keeping the newborn in light for warmth
   c. Consultation with a neonatologist
   d. Careful management of oxygen exposure and periodic eye exams

   Answer: d

5. **In reviewing care guidelines for the child with tympanostomy tubes in place, the nurse informs the parents that the child**
   a. Should be restricted in fluid intake during the first 48 hours after surgery
   b. May go swimming if he wears ear plugs and does not go under water
   c. Must be placed on a soft diet for 10 days following surgery
   d. Will have yellow-green drainage as a result of the tube placement

   Answer: b

6. **The child with frequent and recurrent otitis media may have a delay in**
   a. Speech and language development
   b. Physical growth
   c. Adjustment to school
   d. Sinus development

Answer: a

7. **When treating the child with epistaxis, the nurse determines that the bleeding is anterior, and positions the child**
   a. Prone with one pillow under the head
   b. In a side-lying position
   c. Upright with the head tilted forward
   d. Upright with the head tilted back

Answer: c

8. **Following treatment for an episode of epistaxis, the nurse reviews discharge instructions with parents, which include**
   a. Avoiding cold drinks for 3 days
   b. Warm packs to the nose three times a day
   c. Sleeping without a pillow for 48 hours
   d. Avoiding bending and stooping for 3 days

Answer: d

9. **In order to assist in thinning thick secretions, the nurse instructs the parents of a toddler child with a stuffed nose to**
   a. Place the child in front of a humidifier
   b. Encourage intake of favorite fluids
   c. Feed the child citrus fruits
   d. Place saline-soaked cotton packing in nostrils

Answer: b

10. **The nurse stresses the importance of having the child with strep throat complete the 10-day course of antibiotics prescribed because**
    a. Untreated streptococcal infections may lead to rheumatic fever
    b. Otitis media is also present
    c. The palatine tonsils are enlarged
    d. The child is so ill

Answer: a

11. **In caring for the child who has had a tonsillectomy, the most appropriate nursing diagnosis is high risk for fluid volume deficit related to**
    a. The surgical procedure
    b. Postoperative complications
    c. Reluctance to swallow due to pain
    d. Lack of healing due to bleeding

Answer: c

12. **An important nursing intervention for a post-tonsillectomy child who is high risk for fluid volume deficit is to**
    a. Maintain an intravenous line until the child is taking oral fluids
    b. Avoid irritating the surgical site with hot liquids
    c. Observe the child for signs of discomfort
    d. Observe the child for signs of hemorrhage

Answer: a

13. **When planning activities for the child with visual impairments, it is important for the nurse to remember that**
    a. The sense of smell may also be affected
    b. Socialization skills are underdeveloped
    c. The child should be allowed to play independently
    d. Both fine and gross motor skills may be delayed

Answer: d

14. **Following tonsillectomy surgery, children will typically develop referred pain in the**
    a. Jaw
    b. Eyes
    c. Ear
    d. Nose

Answer: c

15. **When a child has congenital strabismus, the treatment of choice is to**
    a. Apply a patch to the affected eye
    b. Apply a patch to the good eye
    c. Promote use of shaded glasses during daytime
    d. Apply a thin film of antibiotic ointment to the affected eye

Answer: b

16. **A test which is used to assess hearing of various pitches and intensities of sound using earphones is called a**

a. Myringotomy
b. Tympanogram
c. Audiogram
d. Decibel test

Answer: c

17. **If a child communicates by reading lips, the nurse can obtain the child's visual attention by**
    a. Lightly touching the child
    b. Speaking loudly and slowly
    c. Using simple sentences
    d. Clapping the child on the shoulder or arm

Answer: a

18. **In communicating with a hearing-impaired child, the nurse uses hand positions as she speaks to allow the child to see the sound. This technique is called**
    a. Signing
    b. Lip-reading
    c. Cued speech
    d. Gesturing

Answer: c

19. **In the normal visually related developmental milestones, the nurse can expect an infant to pick up a small piece of finger food using a pincer grasp by age**
    a. 7 months
    b. 9 months
    c. 10 months
    d. 12 months

Answer: a

20. **The nurse instructs the mother of an infant with a plugged lacrimal duct to**
    a. Rinse the affected eye with half-strength hydrogen peroxide every 4 hours
    b. Massage the tear duct every 4 hours while the infant is awake
    c. Place a patch over the affected eye during the day
    d. Apply a moist dressing to the eye during the night

Answer: b

21. **During a vision screening, the nurse assesses a child who squints to improve distance vision. This condition is called**
    a. Retinopathy
    b. Myopia
    c. Hyperopia
    d. Astigmatism

Answer: b

22. **During a vision screening, the nurse notes that a child has difficulty focusing in on nearby objects. This condition is called**
    a. Hyperopia
    b. Myopia
    c. Astigmatism
    d. Retinopathy

Answer: a

23. **In assessing the eyes of a 1-month-old infant, the nurse notes visual impairment when the**
    a. Infant blinks greater than 10 times per minute
    b. Eyes have a dull, vacant stare
    c. Infant does not respond to voice
    d. Infant follows the penlight with both eyes

Answer: b

24. **In the event that a child splashes a chemical into the eye, the emergency medical treatment involves**
    a. Transporting the child to the hospital immediately for irrigations
    b. Inverting the upper lid over the lower lid to remove the chemical
    c. Irrigating the eye for 15 to 30 minutes, and then transporting to the hospital
    d. Wiping the eye with a soft, saline-soaked cloth

Answer: c

25. **When a child gets a foreign body on the surface of the eye, it can be removed best by**
    a. Rinsing the eye with half-strength boric acid
    b. Gently rubbing the eye with a soft cloth
    c. Using a tweezer to remove the object
    d. Closing the upper lid over the lower lid

Answer: d

18

ALTERATIONS IN NEUROLOGIC FUNCTION

1. In assessing the neurologic status of a young child, the nurse notes that the child responds to a needle stick, but not to the touch of the hand. These findings are indicative of
   a. Confusion
   b. Delirium
   c. Stupor
   d. Coma

   Answer: c

2. An assessment tool which the nurse uses to compare baseline and subsequent levels of consciousness to evaluate improvement or deterioration in condition is
   a. The Glasgow Coma Scale
   b. a CT scan
   c. An encephalopathy
   d. The Beck Inventory

   Answer: a

3. In an infant, bulging fontanels, widened sutures, dilated scalp veins, and a high-pitched, cat-like cry are
   a. Related to an ineffective breathing pattern
   b. Early signs of increased intracranial pressure
   c. Late signs of hypertension
   d. Indicative of a decreased level of consciousness

   Answer: b

4. The progression of development in fine and gross motor skills in early childhood is a result of the
   a. Stimulation a child receives from parents
   b. Myelination process
   c. Demyelination process
   d. Nutritional intake of the child

   Answer: b

5. In the child with an altered level of consciousness, difficulty in swallowing secretions or absence of a gag reflex alerts the nurse to a need for
   a. Intubation
   b. Suctioning
   c. Increased fluids
   d. Oxygen by mask

   Answer: a

6. A continuous seizure that lasts more than 30 minutes or a series of seizures during which consciousness is not regained is referred to as
   a. Status epilepticus
   b. Self-limiting epilepsy
   c. Tonic-clonic seizure
   d. Absence seizure

   Answer: a

7. **During a seizure in a 7-year-old child, a bite block should not be forced between the teeth because**
   a. This action is considered child abuse
   b. A jaw thrust has not been performed
   c. Permanent teeth may be broken
   d. Shedding deciduous teeth may be aspirated

Answer: d

8. **When assessing a child who has meningitis, the nurse notes resistance as the child's leg is extended at the knee. This reaction is termed a positive**
   a. Opisthotonic sign
   b. Kernig sign
   c. Brudzinski sign
   d. Meningeal sign

Answer: b

9. **When assessing a 10-month-old female who has meningitis, the nurse notes that the child flexes her knees when the nurse flexes the child's head. This finding is referred to as positive**
   a. Opisthotonic sign
   b. Kernig sign
   c. Brudzinski sign
   d. Meningeal sign

Answer: c

10. **In caring for the child who has bacterial meningitis, the nurse initiates a diagnosis for high risk for thermoregulation related to infection. The expected outcome is**
    a. Body temperature is normal within 48 to 72 hours
    b. Body temperature decreases or returns to normal
    c. Antypyretics are effective
    d. Child recovers quickly

Answer: b

11. **In caring for infants who have bacterial meningitis, it is important to measure the head circumference daily because**

   a. Decreasing head circumference may indicate shrinkage of the brain
   b. Of the need to reduce the incidence of neurologic sequelae
   c. Water retention can result in SIADH
   d. Increasing head circumference may indicate subdural effusion or hydrocephalus

Answer: d

12. **Prior to discharge from the hospital, it is important to instruct the parents of a child who had Reye's syndrome that**
    a. There is a definite link between this syndrome and aspirin
    b. All over-the-counter medicines should be checked for the presence of aspirin compound
    c. They should have sought health care sooner
    d. Their child will have neurolgic sequelae

Answer: b

13. **When assessing a child who has encephalitis, it is important to obtain information about**
    a. Recent immunizations, insect bites, and travel
    b. Exposure to oral polio vaccine or to injectable polio vaccine
    c. Recent use of antibiotics
    d. Recent use of antiviral agents

Answer: a

14. **To prevent tetanus in the child who has stepped on a rusty nail, the nurse administers**
    a. Human tetanus immune globulin
    b. Tetanus toxoid
    c. Human tetanus immune globulin and tetanus toxoid
    d. Immune globulin

Answer: b

15. **In the preoperative period, the hospitalized child who has hydrocephalus is given frequent small feedings and "burped" often during feedings because the child**
    a. Has a large, heavy head
    b. Has respiratory problems
    c. Is immobile
    d. Is prone to vomiting

Answer: d

16. A pertinent nursing diagnosis for a child with cerebral palsy is altered nutrition less than body requirements related to
    a. Delayed neuromuscular development
    b. Neuromuscular impairment
    c. Poor sucking and impaired swallowing and chewing
    d. Dependence on others

Answer: c

17. It is imperative that the nurse caring for a child who has a head injury assess the child frequently for signs of ICP because
    a. If untreated, irreversible brain damage may result
    b. Contrecoup injury may occur
    c. Hypoxia may occur
    d. At this time, initial cellular damage can result

Answer: a

18. In teaching the parents of a child with myoclonic seizures about nutritional therapy, the nurse discusses the following diet:
    a. High-protein, low-fat diet
    b. High-fat, low-protein, and low-carbohydrate diet
    c. High-carbohydrate, high-protein and high-fat diet
    d. High-fat and high-carbohydrate diet

Answer: b

19. When a child states that he "felt funny" right before a seizure occurred, the nurse notes the seizure was preceded by an
    a. Aura
    b. Electromagnetic field
    c. Allergic response
    d. Amnesia episode

Answer: a

20. The number one priority nursing intervention during status epilepticus is to
    a. Monitor vital signs
    b. Maintain a patent airway
    c. Protect the child from injury
    d. Manage thermoregulation

Answer: b

21. The infant with bacterial meningitis may assume an opisthotonic position to relieve discomfort. This position is characterized by
    a. A lateral side-lying position with the legs drawn up
    b. Supination of the hands
    c. Dorsiflexion of the feet
    d. Hyperextension of the head and neck

Answer: d

22. The most common neurologic impairment associated with bacterial meningitis in children is
    a. Peripheral neuropathy
    b. Loss of taste
    c. Hearing loss
    d. Visual impairment

Answer: c

23. When working with a child with bacterial meningitis, the nurse can promote a safe return to normal thermoregulation by using the following intervention:
    a. Use of hyperthermia blanket
    b. Use of hypothermia blanket
    c. Administer aspirin as ordered
    d. Submerge the child in a cool water bath

Answer: b

24. Diagnosis of Reye's Syndrome is usually made in stage III of the disease in which the child
    a. Becomes comatose
    b. Is anxious, fearful, and confused
    c. Has severe nausea and vomiting
    d. Demonstrates hyperactive reflexes

Answer: a

25. During the recovery stages of Guillain-Barré syndrome, the priority nursing management for prevention of complications is
    a. Nutritional support for weight gain
    b. Recovery of lost strength
    c. Emotional support for child and parents
    d. Promotion of socialization

Answer: b

19

ALTERATIONS IN MUSCULOSKELETAL FUNCTION

1. **The infant born with metatarsus adductus exhibits a characteristic**
   a. Inward turning of the forefoot
   b. Downward flexion of the foot
   c. Outward turning of the forefoot
   d. Upward flexion of the foot

   Answer: a

2. **The nurse instructs parents of a child with a newly applied cast to elevate the extremity to**
   a. Speed the drying of the cast
   b. Increase venous return
   c. Decrease irritation of cast edges
   d. Improve comfort level

   Answer: b

3. **The nurse instructs the mother of an infant with a club foot to make an appointment for recasting every 2 weeks because of**
   a. Soiling to the casted foot
   b. The need to reposition the foot in the cast
   c. The need for X-rays
   d. Growth of the infant

   Answer: d

4. **The purpose for performing neurovascular checks on an infant following surgical intervention for a club foot is to monitor**
   a. Positioning of the foot
   b. Movement of the leg
   c. Color, temperature, and movement of the toes
   d. Pain to the casted extremity

   Answer: c

5. **The nurse instructs the parents of a child who must wear a brace to toughen up the sensitive skin areas with the use of**
   a. Powder
   b. Alcohol
   c. Lotion
   d. Betadine

   Answer: b

6. **The symptom of partial dislocation of the hip in a child with congenital dislocation is referred to as**
   a. Subluxation
   b. Genu valgum
   c. Genu varum
   d. Club foot

   Answer: a

7. **In assessing an infant for developmental dysplasia of the hip, a nurse identifies its presence by noting**
   a. Excessive abduction on the affected side
   b. A negative Ortolani maneuver
   c. Asymmetrical gluteal folds
   d. Adduction on the affected side

   Answer: c

8. The nurse teaches the mother of a child who must wear a Pavlik harness to apply the device. In evaluating the effectiveness of the teaching plan, the nurse has the mother
   a. Verbally describe its use
   b. Explain its application
   c. Evaluated by a home health agency
   d. Apply it to the infant

Answer: d

9. The primary nurse caring for a child in a spica cast needs to assess the patient every day for
   a. Hyperreflexia
   b. Anorexia
   c. Hydration
   d. Constipation

Answer: d

10. In obtaining a nursing history, sudden severe pain and the inability to bear weight on a lower extremity are frequent complaints verbalized by an adolescent with
    a. Legg-Calvé-Perthes disease
    b. Fracture femur
    c. Slipped capital femoral epiphysis
    d. Skeletal tuberculosis

Answer: c

11. The most appropriate nursing diagnosis for the child with a slipped capital femoral epiphysis is
    a. High risk for infection
    b. Impaired physical mobility related to non-weight-bearing treatment regimen
    c. High risk for noncompliance related to prolonged treatment program
    d. Activity intolerance related to brace wear

Answer: b

12. After treatment for slipped capital femoral epiphysis, the adolescent needs to understand that follow-up visits are necessary until
    a. After weight bearing on the affected extremity begins
    b. The surgical site is healed completely
    c. Weight is within the normal range for age
    d. The epiphyseal plates are closed

Answer: d

13. For the child with a moderate form of scoliosis, treatment focuses on
    a. Bracing
    b. Stretching
    c. Surgery
    d. Exercising

Answer: a

14. In performing a scoliosis screening, the nurse recognizes that the most common classic sign of scoliosis is
    a. A limp
    b. Pain in the hip
    c. Truncal asymmetry
    d. Leg length discrepancy

Answer: c

15. The adolescent with scoliosis who is in a Milwaukee brace should know that this device needs to be worn
    a. During waking hours only
    b. Only at night
    c. When discomfort occurs
    d. At all times

Answer: d

16. The parents of a child diagnosed with scoliosis ask the nurse if there are any alternate active treatments for scoliosis other than the Milwaukee brace. The nurse discusses
    a. Stretching
    b. Electrical stimulation
    c. Surgery
    d. Exercise

Answer: b

17. The postoperative nursing management of a child who has had a Harrington rod inserted and a spinal fusion done requires
    a. Bed rest
    b. Use of a Milwaukee brace
    c. Prolonged immobilization
    d. Electrical stimulation

Answer: c

18. A school nurse should begin screening children for scoliosis in the
    a. Third grade
    b. Fifth grade
    c. Seventh grade
    d. Ninth grade

    Answer: b

19. The nurse reviewing limitations placed on an adolescent who has had surgery to correct scoliosis stresses maintaining these restrictions for
    a. 1 to 3 months
    b. 3 to 6 months
    c. 6 to 9 months
    d. 9 to 12 months

    Answer: c

20. Postural lordosis is a characteristic finding in toddlers, but nurses need to reassure parents that it will disappear by
    a. The preschool years
    b. School age
    c. Adolescence
    d. Adulthood

    Answer: b

21. Pain in the adolescent after surgery for scoliosis can best be controlled by administering medications
    a. Around the clock
    b. According to the Q4H schedule
    c. Whenever requested
    d. After a pain assessment

    Answer: a

22. During the first 2 days following corrective surgery for scoliosis, how frequently should a nurse encourage active and passive range-of-motion exercises?
    a. Q2H
    b. Q4H
    c. Q6H
    d. Q8H

    Answer: a

23. In providing care to a toddler with osteomyelitis of the left knee, a critical nursing intervention is
    a. Forcing fluids
    b. Providing a high-protein diet
    c. Positioning Q4H
    d. Immobilization

    Answer: d

24. Children with muscular dystrophy compensate for weak lower extremities by using the upper extremity muscles to raise themselves to a standing position. This is called the
    a. Barlow test
    b. Ortolani maneuver
    c. Allis sign
    d. Gower maneuver

    Answer: d

25. In preparing parents for the discharge of their toddler who was treated for osteomyelitis, a nurse needs to emphasize the importance of
    a. Providing a high-protein, high-fiber diet
    b. Completing the course of antibiotics
    c. Maintaining bedrest
    d. Giving large amounts of liquids

    Answer: b

20

ALTERATIONS IN
ENDOCRINE FUNCTION

1. The child newly diagnosed with diabetes exhibits symptoms of extreme thirst, stating, "I drink gallons of water and can't seem to quench my thirst." This is referred to as
   a. Polyphagia
   b. Polydypsia
   c. Polyuria
   d. Aquaemia

Answer: b

2. In plotting the height of a 12-month-old, a nurse finds she is three standard deviations below the mean height for her age, which may indicate a deficiency in
   a. Cortisol
   b. Growth hormone
   c. Androgens
   d. Thyroxine

Answer: b

3. In psychosocial dwarfism, a child is removed from a stressful environment, provided with a normal dietary intake, and experiences dramatic catch-up growth as a result of the restoration of
   a. Adrenal secretion
   b. Thyroid secretion
   c. Hypothalamic function
   d. Pituitary secretion

Answer: d

4. In caring for a child with hypopituitarism, the nurse teaches parents how to administer the missing growth hormone preparation by instructing how to give
   a. Rectal suppositories
   b. Subcutaneous injections
   c. Intramuscular injections
   d. Intravenous medication

Answer: b

5. When a child with diabetes insipidus is given a water deprivation test, it results in
   a. Increased weight gain
   b. Unchanged specific gravity
   c. Excessive protein excretion
   d. Accumulation of ammonia

Answer: b

6. In the presence of true ADH deficiency, a nurse needs to teach parents how to administer desmopressin
   a. Intravenously
   b. Orally
   c. Subcutaneously
   d. Intranasally

Answer: d

7. In precocious puberty, breast development with pubic hair occurs as early as age
   a. 6 years
   b. 8 years
   c. 10 years
   d. 12 years
   Answer: b

8. When a synthetic thyroid preparation is prescribed for the infant with hypo-thyroidism, the nurse informs parents that the child will be on the medication
   a. Until after preschool years
   b. Until age 10 years
   c. Through adolescence
   d. Throughout adulthood
   Answer: d

9. Signs and symptoms of Graves' disease, such as tachycardia, tumors, excessive perspiration, and emotional lability, are caused by
   a. High thyroid hormone levels
   b. A thyroid adenoma
   c. A hyperactive sympathetic nervous system
   d. Immunoglobulins
   Answer: c

10. In order to promote the caloric intake of an adolescent with hyperthyroidism, the nurse encourages the intake of
    a. Three balanced meals a day
    b. Five or six moderate meals a day
    c. Midmorning, afternoon, and evening supplements
    d. Four or five small meals each day
    Answer: b

11. In helping parents to understand the overproduction of parathyroid hormone, the nurse explains the effect of an increase in the reabsorption of
    a. Phosphorus
    b. Sodium
    c. Calcium
    d. Potassium
    Answer: c

12. The postoperative nursing care of a child who has had a craniotomy for primary hyperparathyroidism includes the frequent monitoring of
    a. Phosphorus levels
    b. Calcium levels
    c. Potassium levels
    d. Sodium levels
    Answer: b

13. The clinical manifestations of hypercalcemia in a child include nausea, vomiting, behavioral changes, abdominal pain, and
    a. Hypotonia
    b. Weight gain
    c. Apnea
    d. Bradycardia
    Answer: a

14. For the child who needs cortisol replacement, the nurse teaches parents to administer the cortisol
    a. Early in the morning
    b. During the noon meal
    c. During the evening meal
    d. Prior to bedtime
    Answer: a

15. In some children with congenital adrenal hyperplasia, the cause of the excessive renal excretion of salt is a deficiency in
    a. Parathyroid hormone
    b. Aldosterone synthesis
    c. Antidiuretic hormone
    d. Thyroid
    Answer: b

16. In preparing feedings for a newborn who has partial or complete 21-hydroxylase enzyme deficiency with congenital adrenal hyperplasia, the nurse recognizes the importance of adding the following to the formula:
    a. Calcium
    b. Potassium
    c. Glucose
    d. Sodium chloride
    Answer: d

17. When asking about future child-bearing possibilities for their newborn with ambiguous genitalia, parents should be advised that after reconstructive surgery
    a. It depends on her hormonal status
    b. It may not be possible
    c. All organs are functional
    d. She will be sterile

Answer: c

18. Preoperatively, an important nursing intervention to implement in caring for a child who has a pheochromocytoma is
    a. Forcing fluids
    b. Providing a high-calorie protein diet
    c. Placing him on seizure precautions
    d. Monitoring his specific gravity

Answer: c

19. The most objective measurement of glycemia control over a period of time is
    a. Daily urine for glucose
    b. 2-hour postprandial blood sugar
    c. Blood glucose monitoring
    d. Glucosylated hemoglobin

Answer: d

20. In teaching the adolescent administration of insulin, the nurse reviews the fact that NPH insulin peaks in
    a. 2 to 4 hours
    b. 4 to 8 hours
    c. 6 to 12 hours
    d. 12 to 24 hours

Answer: c

21. In obtaining a growth history from parents of a 10-year-old who is being worked up for Turner's syndrome, her parents tell the nurse her rate of growth seemed to be normal until she was
    a. 1 year old
    b. 3 years old
    c. 5 years old
    d. 7 years old

Answer: b

22. In treating a girl with Turner's syndrome, initial therapy consists of low-dose
    a. Estrogen
    b. Follicle-stimulating hormone
    c. Androgens
    d. Growth hormone

Answer: a

23. Children who are either short in stature or tall for their age may have a problem that is related to
    a. Teasing
    b. Learning disorders
    c. Overprotectiveness
    d. Self-image

Answer: d

24. During fetal development, the endocrine system is responsible for
    a. Sexual differentiation
    b. Growth and development
    c. Development of reproductive systems
    d. Maintaining optimal hormonal levels

Answer: a

25. Puberty occurs when the gonads secrete increased amounts of
    a. Estrogen and aldosterone
    b. Testosterone and prolactin
    c. Androgens and follicle-stimulating hormone
    d. Estrogen and testosterone

Answer: d

21

ALTERATIONS IN
SKIN INTEGRITY

1. A school-age child who has pediculosis capitus asks you why her bedding and clothing must be changed and laundered daily. You explain that although lice can survive for only 48 hours away from a human host,
   a. They have a life span of 30 days
   b. Nits that are shed may hatch 8 to 10 days later
   c. Nits will be killed by the first pediculicide
   d. Lice are transmitted by direct contact

   Answer: b

2. You are assessing a child's skin. You discover several secondary lesions that have a dried residue of serum. They are referred to as
   a. Lichenifications
   b. Scales
   c. Keloids
   d. Crusts

   Answer: d

3. During an assessment of a 12-year-old, you find thin flakes of exfoliated epidermis. These lesions are termed
   a. Lichenifications
   b. Scales
   c. Keloids
   d. Crusts

   Answer: b

4. The nurse instructs the mother of a baby with diaper rash to discontinue using disposable baby wipes because
   a. The alcohol content in this product is sufficient to exacerbate the condition
   b. The alcohol in the wipes reacts with the urine to form ammonia
   c. This product has a drying effect
   d. There is no contraindication to using this product

   Answer: a

5. When providing nursing intervention for the infant who has seborrheic dermatitis, the nurse teaches parents to prevent further episodes by
   a. The use of 0.5% hydrocortisone cream
   b. Keeping the scalp clean
   c. Changing soiled diapers immediately
   d. Washing the area with mild soap and water and patting dry

   Answer: b

6. In a 6-month-old infant, you made a nursing diagnosis of impaired skin integrity related to open vesicles and lesions. An important teaching point to prevent scratching and reduce the chance of secondary infection is to advise parents to

a. Avoid using harsh or performed soaps
b. Apply 1% hydrocortisone to affected lesions for 4 to 5 days
c. Place clean cotton gloves or socks over infant's hands
d. Use colloidal baths

Answer: c

7. **Impetigo is easily spread from child to child in close quarters because the lesions are contagious**
   a. Until treatment is completed
   b. Prior to formation
   c. For the first 3 days of treatment
   d. For the first 24 hours after formation

Answer: d

8. **When assessing a child who has a dermatophytosis, it is important to ask if**
   a. The child is taking antibiotics
   b. The child has thrush
   c. There are household pets
   d. Occlusive clothing is being worn

Answer: c

9. **A father asks you why his son's cellulitis is being treated so aggressively. The nurse explains that, if untreated,**
   a. Osteomyelitis can result
   b. The infection will spread
   c. Inflammation will occur
   d. Vital signs will change

Answer: a

10. **An appropriate goal for the nursing diagnosis of body image disturbance related to visible facial lesions is that the adolescent will**
    a. Show increased confidence, as evidenced by involvement in activities
    b. Freely discuss concerns and fears
    c. Keep a personal diary for 1 week
    d. Demonstrate increased self-confidence and self-esteem

Answer: d

11. **Adolescents with acne who are being treated with vitamin A preparations need to be aware that**

a. They should not use cosmetics that have a greasy base
b. Flare-ups will occur
c. Their skin may become sensitive to light
d. Treatment is short-term

Answer: c

12. **Children who have minor burns generally are not hospitalized. Parents are instructed about fluid needs, diet, and pain management. In order to monitor progress, the child is seen**
    a. Every day for a week
    b. Within 48 hours of treatment
    c. As often as parents deem necessary
    d. At follow-up appointments

Answer: b

13. **Since burn wound care is often a painful procedure, the nurse should administer pain medication**
    a. 15 minutes prior to the procedure
    b. 30 minutes prior to the procedure
    c. 45 minutes prior to the procedure
    d. 60 minutes prior to the procedure

Answer: b

14. **When treating burn patients, whirlpool baths are given not only before debridement, but also to**
    a. Provide a means for daily bathing
    b. Soothe the child and provide relaxation
    c. Increase the child's circulation and speed healing of the burns
    d. Cleanse the wound prior to dressing and remove dead tissue

Answer: c

15. **When assessing a child while taking a burn history, thorough documentation is necessary to**
    a. Rule out child abuse
    b. Determine the depth of the burn
    c. Assess parental anxiety
    d. Discover who is responsible

Answer: a

16. **For the burned child, it is important to assess the level of pain frequently because**
   a. The child needs an outlet for emotions
   b. Changes in location may indicate complications
   c. Vital signs may be affected
   d. Of accompanying joint pain

   Answer: c

17. **The parents of a child with a severe burn injury ask you why debridement is necessary. You explain that this procedure allows**
   a. New epidermis to form
   b. Blisters to be removed
   c. The area to remain sterile
   d. Granulation tissue to form

   Answer: d

18. **The child who has suffered a major burn injury is at high risk for fluid volume excess or deficit related to**
   a. Hypervolemia
   b. Loss of fluid through wounds and/or hemorrhagic loss
   c. Destruction of the skin barrier and traumatized tissue
   d. Edema

   Answer: b

19. **It is important that children with a major burn receive vitamin C supplements because this vitamin aids**
   a. Zinc absorption
   b. Healing
   c. Altered nutrition
   d. Mobility

   Answer: a

20. **Parents often feel guilty about and responsible for their child's major burn injury. When providing them with emotional support, the nurse should help them focus on**
   a. Disfigurement and scarring
   b. Interest and concern
   c. Recovery rather than past actions
   d. Development of trust in the health team

   Answer: c

21. **In helping parents understand the importance of applying sun block to their children when they must be out in the sun, the nurse explains that repeated sunburns can cause**
   a. Permanent scarring and brown spots
   b. Hyperthermia
   c. Inflamed joints
   d. Permanent skin damage and skin cancer

   Answer: d

22. **When treating a child with frostbite, the child complains of tingling during the rewarming phase. The nurse recognizes that**
   a. Sensation is returning
   b. Oxygen therapy is indicated
   c. Rewarming must be done more slowly
   d. Cellular damage has occurred

   Answer: a

23. **The nurse working in an urgent care clinic assesses a child who has just been bitten by a dog. The nurse checks the child's immunization record to determine if the child needs**
   a. Rabies immune globulin
   b. Antirabies serum
   c. A tetanus booster
   d. Treatment

   Answer: c

24. **A father asks you how to determine if a brown spider is a brown recluse spider. The nurse responds that the recluse spider**
   a. Leaves red fang marks at the site of the bite
   b. Has a fiddle-shaped marking on its head
   c. Causes a stinging sensation as it bites
   d. Is smaller than other brown spiders

   Answer: b

25. **Most commercial insect repellents contain diethyltoluamide (DEET). Parents should avoid overuse of these products, especially with infants and young children, because**
   a. DEET is absorbed quickly
   b. Diarrhea can result with repeated applications
   c. Skin injury can occur
   d. Toxic encephalopathy has been reported following repeated use

   Answer: d

22

ALTERATIONS IN PSYCHOSOCIAL FUNCTION

1. **The nurse caring for an autistic adolescent who is particularly aggressive and self-abusive maintains a safe environment for the teenager by**
   a. Restraining the teenager in bed
   b. Trying to keep the environment consistent, by not moving objects
   c. Monitoring the adolescent at all times
   d. Placing a bike helmet on the teen's head and mitts on the teen's hands

   Answer: d

2. **Therapeutic interventions and communications are based on the principle that**
   a. The child and family can reduce the impact of stressors
   b. Parents react to children's behavior
   c. Any unlearned behavior can be unlearned
   d. The feelings behind the behavior must be examined

   Answer: d

3. **One therapeutic strategy that the nurse can use when working with children who have psychosocial disorders is**
   a. Individual play
   b. Therapeutic play
   c. Play therapy
   d. Group therapy

   Answer: c

4. **When using principles of behavior modification, the nurse recognizes that the therapy is more effective if attention is given to**
   a. Consistency
   b. Conditioning
   c. Guided imagery
   d. Relaxation

   Answer: a

5. **When used in conjunction with a thorough history and appropriate psychological testing information, art can be employed to**
   a. Reveal problems on a fantasy level
   b. Guide therapy
   c. Provide a safe, supportive environment
   d. Form a developmental perspective

   Answer: b

6. **In discussing the disease of autism, the nurse explains that the cause is**
   a. Brain dysfunction
   b. Unknown
   c. Low IQ
   d. Birth trauma

   Answer: b

7. When caring for an autistic child who is hospitalized, the nurse decreases environmental stimuli because the child may interpret "ordinary sounds" as
   a. Louder, more frightening, and overwhelming
   b. Signals to become self-abusive
   c. Music for dancing
   d. Nonverbal communication
   Answer: a

8. Parents ask you if their child who has attention deficit hyperactivity disorder (ADHD) will ever gain control over impulses. The nurse explains that
   a. With medication, the child will improve
   b. The child will always have behavior problems, especially in school
   c. Attention span lengthens and impulse control improves during adolescence
   d. By adulthood, the child will be normal
   Answer: c

9. A mother asks the nurse how she can reduce specific behaviors in her child who has ADHD. The nurse discusses the use of
   a. Play therapy
   b. Guided imagery
   c. Hypnosis
   d. Behavior modification
   Answer: d

10. The preterm infant needs frequent, thorough neurologic and developmental assessments, especially during the first year of life, because of the risk for
    a. Below normal cognitive development
    b. Cerebral palsy
    c. Hydrocephaly
    d. Microcephaly
    Answer: a

11. Parents of a child recently diagnosed as mentally retarded express to the nurse their fears that they will be unable to afford special education for the child. The nurse discusses

   a. Availability of special programs
   b. Provisions of PL94-142 and PL99-457
   c. Application of results of functional assessment
   d. Ways to teach the child activities of daily living
   Answer: b

12. In the anorectic child, a nursing diagnosis of high risk for fluid volume deficit is related to inadequate fluid intake or
    a. Distorted beliefs about fluid requirements
    b. Overuse of laxatives and diuretics
    c. Absence of subcutaneous fat
    d. Refusal to eat
    Answer: b

13. As part of nursing interventions, the clinical nurse specialist teaches depressed children positive coping strategies. Examples of effective techniques are
    a. Play therapy and art therapy
    b. Guided imagery and relaxation
    c. Hypnosis and behavior modification
    d. Family and group therapy
    Answer: b

14. An adolescent with anorexia is receiving TPN. As part of the assessment, the nurse observes the teen for the following complications:
    a. Abdominal distension, constipation, or diarrhea
    b. Bizarre eating and drinking behaviors
    c. Circulatory overload, hyperglycemia, and hypoglycemia
    d. Hypertension and tachycardia
    Answer: c

15. Bulimic adolescents lose their ability to respond to normal cues of hunger and satiety as a result of
    a. Repeated practice of the binge-purge cycle
    b. Repeated induced vomiting several times a day
    c. Overuse of laxatives
    d. Poor body image and dysfunctional family dynamics
    Answer: a

16. **In order to evaluate the effect of antidepressants on a child's mood, it is essential that the nurse**
    a. Document resultant behavior
    b. Teach positive coping strategies
    c. Identify events that precipitate feelings of help-lessness
    d. Be supportive

    Answer: a

17. **The nurse monitors the bulimic patients for at least a half-hour following meals to ensure that they**
    a. Can keep the food down
    b. Do not hide or give away their food
    c. Do not attempt purging activities
    d. Are in electrolyte balance

    Answer: c

18. **In general, substance abuse in children and adolescents represents**
    a. Complying with peer pressure
    b. The need to excel intellectually and socially
    c. Lack of self-esteem
    d. A maladaptive coping response to stress

    Answer: d

19. **Many risk factors for suicide exist in children and adolescents. The most common precursor to adolescent suicide is**
    a. Pregnancy
    b. Drug use or abuse
    c. Poor health
    d. Depression

    Answer: d

20. **When eliciting a history from parents about child abuse–related concerns, the nurse should begin**
    a. By stating that abuse is suspected
    b. By interviewing each parent separately
    c. With nonthreatening topics
    d. With observation of parent-child interactions

    Answer: c

21. **In doing a preliminary abdominal assessment of the adolescent girl with anorexia, the nurse will most likely note**
    a. A soft, nontender abdomen
    b. Hyperactive bowel sounds
    c. Complaints of abdominal discomfort
    d. A flat, muscular abdomen

    Answer: c

22. **As a result of protein-calorie malnutrition, the adolescent with anorexia will develop**
    a. Ketoacidosis
    b. Hypertension and tachycardia
    c. Hyperglycemia and vertigo
    d. Leukopenia and hypoglycemia

    Answer: d

23. **The adolescent with anorexia expends a great deal of energy in vigorous exercise, up to**
    a. 30 minutes daily
    b. 1 hour daily
    c. 2 hours daily
    d. 4 hours daily

    Answer: d

24. **When performing a physical assessment of the bulimic adolescent, the nurse will most likely note that the enamel of the teeth are**
    a. Badly eroded
    b. Chipped
    c. Stained
    d. Bubbled

    Answer: a

25. **A child with schizophrenia will display characteristic behaviors which include**
    a. Euphoric affect and concrete thought processes
    b. Flat affect and flight of ideas
    c. Charm and wit
    d. Social attachment and dependency on others

    Answer: b

AUDIO-VISUAL RESOURCES

Abbott Scientific Products Division
820 Mission Street
South Pasadena, California 91030

AIMS Media
6901 Woodley Avenue
Van Nuys, California 91406

American Broadcasting Company
1313 Avenue of the Americas
New York, New York 10019

American Cancer Society
777 Third Avenue
New York, New York 100 17
(212) 371-2900

American Journal of Nursing Co.
555 West 57th Street
New York, New York 10019-2961
1-800-CALL AJN

American Lung Association
1740 Broadway
New York, New York 10019

American Red Cross
Los Angeles Chapter
2700 Wiltshire Boulevard
Los Angeles, California 90010

Association for the Care of Children's Health
3615 Wisconsin Avenue, N.W.
Washington, D.C. 20016
(202) 244-1801

Career Aids
20417 Nordhoff Street
Department HA
Chatsworth, California 91311
(818) 341-2535

Carle Medical Communications
5 10 West Main Street
Urbana, Illinois 61801

Child, Youth and Family Services
1741 Silverlake Boulevard
Los Angeles, California 90026

Churchill Films
660 North Robertson Boulevard
Los Angeles, California 90069
(213) 657-5110

Concept Media
P.O. Box 19542
Irvine, CA 92623-9542
(800) 233-7078

Cutter Biological
Cutter Laboratories, Inc.
Berkeley, California 94710

Cystic Fibrosis Foundation
6000 Executive Boulevard
Suite 309
Rockville, Maryland 20852

Encyclopedia Britannica Educational Corporation
425 North Michigan Avenue
Chicago, Illinois 60611
1-800-558-6968

Fairview General Hospital
1801 Lorain Avenue
Cleveland, Ohio 44111

Fanlight Productions
47 Halifax Street
Boston, Massachusetts 02130
(800) 937-4113

Film Fair Communications
10900 Ventura Boulevard, Box 1728
Studio City, California 91604
(818) 985-0244

Filmmaker's Library
133 East 58th Street
New York, New York 10022
(212) 355-6545

Films for the Humanities and Sciences
P.O. Box 2053
Princeton, New Jersey 08543-2053
(800) 257-5126

Guidance Associates
Communications Park
Box 3000
Mount Kisco, New York 10549
1-800-431-2266

Health Sciences Consortium
201 Silver Cedar Court
Chapel Hill, North Carolina 27514
(919) 942-8731

Human Relations Media
Room GC
175 Tompkins Avenue
Pleasantville, New York 10570
(914) 769-7496

Insight Media
2162 Broadway
New York, New York 10024-6620
(800) 233-9910

J. B. Lippincott Company
P.O. Box 1600
Hagerstown, Maryland 21741-9910
(800) 777-2295

Johnson and Johnson
Mead Johnson and Company
2404 West Pennsylvania Street
Evansville, Indiana 47721

Kid's Corner
2927 North Tejon Street
Colorado Springs, Colorado 80907
(303) 475-2499

March of Dimes Birth Defects Foundation
1275 Mamaroneck Avenue
White Plains, New York 10605
(914) 428-7100

M.D.A. TV
M. D. Anderson Hospital
6723 Bertner Avenue, Mail Box 74
Houston, Texas 77030
(713) 792-7287

MedCom/Trainex - Nasco Health Care Educational
12601 Industry Street
P. 0. Box 3225
Garden Grove, California 92642
(714) 891-1443

Medical Electronic Educational Services, Inc.
Teaching Films, Inc.
930 Pitner Avenue
Evanston, Illinois 60202
(312) 326-6700

NAPHT, Inc. New York Chapter
c/o Mr. Gerald Dessner
220 East 67th Street
New York, New York 10021

National Audio-Visual Center
8700 Edgeworth Drive
Capitol Heights, Maryland 20743
(301) 763-1896

National Foundation for Ileitis and Colitis, Inc.
444 Park Avenue South
New York, New York 10016
(212) 685-3340

National Hemophilia Foundation
35 West 39th Street
New York, New York 10016

National Society to Prevent Blindness
70 Madison Avenue
New York, New York 10016

Network for Continuing Medical Education
Roche Laboratories
c/o Association Sterling Films, Inc.
600 Grand Avenue
Ridgefield, New Jersey 07657

New England Regional Genetics Group (NERGG)
P. 0. Box 670
Mount Desert, Maine 04660
(207) 288-2704

Paul H. Brookes Publishing Company, Inc.
P. 0. Box 10624
Baltimore, Maryland 21285

Prentice-Hall Media
150 White Plains Road
Tarrytown, New York 10591

Public Television Library
475 L'Enfant Plaza, S.W.
Washington, D.C. 20024

Pyramid Film and Video
Box 1048
Santa Monica, California 90406
(213) 828-7577

Rhode Island Office of Refugee Resettlement
600 New London Avenue
Cranston, Rhode Island 02900
(401) 464-2127

Ross Laboratories
Educational Services Department
625 Cleveland Avenue
Columbus, Ohio 43216
(614) 227-3557

Trainex Corporation
P. 0. Box 115
Garden Grove, California 92542

Umbrella Films
60 Blake Road
Brookline, Massachusetts 02146

Universal Education and Visual Arts
Division of Universal City Studios, Inc.
100 Universal City Plaza
Universal City, California 90038

University of Arizona
Biomedical Communications
Health Sciences Center
Tucson, Arizona 85724

University of Kansas Medical Center
Department of Preventive Medicine
4004 Robinson, 3901 Rainbow Boulevard
Kansas City, Kansas 66160
(913) 588-2762

University of Michigan Medical Center
Media Library
Towsley Center for Continuing Medical Education
Box 58
Ann Arbor, Michigan 48109
(313) 763-2074

Vacurnate Corporation
114 West 20th Street
New York, New York 10001